# Cardiology and the
# Cardiovascular System
## *on the move*

# Medicine *on the move*

*Editor-in-chief: Rory Mackinnon*
*Series editors: Sally Keat, Thomas Locke, Andrew Walker and Harriet Walker*

## RECENT AND FORTHCOMING TITLES

Cardiology and the Cardiovascular System on the Move
David Dunleavy, Swati Gupta and Alexandra Marsh, 2015

Clinical Pharmacology and Practical Prescribing on the Move
James Turnbull and Matthew Tate, 2015

Emergency and Acute Medicine on the Move
Naomi Meardon, Shireen Siddiqui, Elena Del Vescovo, Lucy C Peart
and Sherif Hemaya, 2015

Gastroenterology on the Move
Arash Assadsangabi, Lucy Carroll and Andrew Irvine, 2015

Neurology and Clinical Neuroanatomy on the Move
Matthew Tate, Johnathan Cooper-Knock, Zoe Hunter and Elizabeth Wood, 2014

Surgery on the Move
Jenna Morgan, Harriet Walker and Andrew Viggars, 2014

Orthopaedics and Rheumatology on the Move
Terence McLoughlin, Ian Baxter and Nicole Abdul, 2013

Obstetrics, Gynaecology and Women's Health on the Move
Amie Clifford, Claire Kelly, Chris Yau and Sally Hallam, 2012

Psychiatry on the Move
Molly Douglas, Harriet Walker and Helen Casey, 2012

Anaesthesia on the Move
Sally Keat, Simon Bate, Alexander Bown and Sarah Lanham, 2012

Clinical Investigations on the Move
Andrew Walker, Lina Fazlanie and Rory Mackinnon, 2012

Microbiology and Infectious Diseases on the Move
Thomas Locke, Sally Keat, Andrew Walker and Rory Mackinnon, 2012

# Cardiology and the Cardiovascular System
## *on the move*

Authors: Swati Gupta, Alexandra Marsh
and David Dunleavy
Editorial Advisor: Kevin Channer

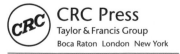

## CRC Press
Taylor & Francis Group
Boca Raton  London  New York

CRC Press is an imprint of the
Taylor & Francis Group, an **informa** business

CRC Press
Taylor & Francis Group
6000 Broken Sound Parkway NW, Suite 300
Boca Raton, FL 33487-2742

Printed on acid-free paper
Version Date: 20151015

International Standard Book Number-13: 978-1-4441-7599-8 (Pack - Book and Ebook)

**Visit the Taylor & Francis Web site at**
**http://www.taylorandfrancis.com**

**and the CRC Press Web site at**
**http://www.crcpress.com**

# Contents

# Preface

Have you ever found cardiology and the physiology of the cardiovascular system overwhelmingly complicated? Have you struggled to recall the basics in a clinical situation? Or are you simply short of time and have exams looming? If so, this concise, practical guide will help you.

Written by doctors for doctors, this book presents information in a wide range of formats including flow charts, boxes, summary tables and colourful diagrams. No matter what your learning style, we hope that you will find the book appealing and easy to read. We think that the innovative style will help you, the reader, to connect with this often feared topic, to learn, understand and even enjoy it, and to apply what you have learned in your clinical practice and in the pressured run-up to final examinations.

In writing the book, we have drawn on our recent personal experience as medical students and junior doctors, and hope this book will offer the less-experienced a portable and practical guide to cardiology that will complement larger reference texts. We hope you find it helpful!

We would like to thank Dr Pankaj Garg, Cardiac MR Research Fellow, University of Leeds, Leeds, who provided us several of the images to this book.

## AUTHORS

**Swati Gupta** MBChB (Hons), BMedSci – CT2 Anaesthetic ACCS Trainee, Cheltenham Hospital, Gloucestershire NHS Foundation Trust, Gloucestershire, UK

**Alexandra Marsh** MBChB (Hons), BMedSci – Foundation Year 2 Doctor, Sheffield Teaching Hospitals, Sheffield, UK

**David Dunleavy** MBChB, BSc – Ophthalmology Spr, York Teaching Hospital NHS Foundation Trust, York, UK

## EDITORIAL ADVISOR

**Kevin Channer** BSc (Hons) MBChB (Hons) MD FRCP – Consultant Cardiologist, Honorary Professor of Cardiovascular Medicine, Sheffield Hallam University, Sheffield, UK

## EDITOR-IN-CHIEF

**Rory Mackinnon** BSc (Hons) MBChB MRCGP – GP Partner, Dr Cloak & Partners, Southwick Health Centre, Sunderland, UK

## SERIES EDITORS

**Sally Keat** MBChB BMedSci MRCP – Core Medical Trainee Year 2 in Barts Health NHS Trust, London, UK

**Thomas Locke** BSc, MBChB, DTM&H, MRCP(UK) – Core Medical Trainee Year 2, Northwick Park Hospital, London Northwest Healthcare London, UK

**Andrew MN Walker** BMedSci MBChB MRCP (London) – British Heart Foundation Clinical Research Fellow and Honorary Specialist Registrar in Cardiology, University of Leeds, UK

# List of abbreviations

- AA: arachidonic acid
- ABG: arterial blood gas
- ACEi: angiotensin-converting enzyme inhibitor
- ACS: acute coronary syndrome
- AF: atrial fibrillation
- AHF: acute heart failure
- ALS: advanced life support
- APTT: activated partial thromboplastin time
- AR: acute regurgitation
- ARB: angiotensin receptor blocker
- ARDS: acute respiratory distress syndrome
- ARVC: arrhythmogenic right ventricular cardiomyopathy
- ARVD: arrhythmogenic right ventricular dysplasia
- AS: aortic valve stenosis
- ASD: atrial septal defect
- AST: aspartate aminotransferase
- AV: atrioventricular
- AVNRT: AV nodal re-entry tachycardia
- AVRT: AV re-entry tachycardia
- AVSD: atrioventricular septal defect
- BMI: body mass index
- BMS: bare-metal stent
- BNP: brain natriuretic peptide
- BP: blood pressure
- CABG: coronary artery bypass graft
- CAD: coronary artery disease
- CCF: congestive cardiac failure
- CCU: coronary care unit
- CHF: chronic heart failure
- CK: creatine kinase
- COPD: chronic obstructive pulmonary disease
- COX: cyclooxygenase
- CPAP: continuous positive airway pressure
- CPVT: catecholaminergic polymorphic ventricular tachycardia
- CRP: C-reactive protein
- CVD: cardiovascular disease
- CXR: plain chest radiograph
- DAPT: Dual Anti-Platelet Therapy
- DES: drug-eluting stent

- ESC: European Society of Cardiology
- ESR: erythrocyte sedimentation rate
- FBC: full blood count
- GRACE: Global Registry for Acute Coronary Events
- GTN: glyceryl trinitrate
- HDL: high-density lipoprotein
- HF: heart failure
- HR: heart rate
- HSTn: high sensitivity troponin
- IABP: intra-aortic balloon pump
- ICD: implantable cardioverter defibrillator
- ILR: implantable loop ECG recorder
- INR: international normalized ratio
- ISDN: isosorbide dinitrate
- ISMN: isosorbide mononitrate
- ITU: intensive treatment unit
- IVDU: intravenous drug user
- JVP: jugular venous pressure
- LA: left atrium
- LAD: left anterior descending artery
- LBBB: left bundle branch block
- LDH: lactate dehydrogenase
- LDL: low-density lipoprotein
- LFT: liver function tests
- LMWH: low-molecular-weight heparin
- LV: left ventricle
- LVEF: left ventricular ejection fraction
- LVH: left ventricular hypertrophy
- LVSF: left ventricular systolic function
- MI: myocardial infarction
- NIV: non-invasive ventilation
- NSTEMI: non-ST segment elevation myocardial infarction
- NSVT: non-sustained ventricular tachycardia
- PCI: percutaneous coronary intervention
- PCWP: pulmonary capillary wedge pressure
- PDA: persistent ductus arteriosus
- PE: pulmonary embolus
- PEA: pulseless electrical activity
- PFO: patent foramen ovale
- PND: paroxysmal nocturnal dyspnoea
- PT: prothrombin time
- PVR: peripheral vascular resistance
- RA: right atrium

- RAAS: renin–angiotensin–aldosterone system
- RBBB: right bundle branch block
- RCA: right coronary artery
- RCC: right coronary cusp
- RVH: right ventricular hypertrophy
- RV: right ventricle
- SBP: systolic blood pressure
- SLE: systemic lupus erythematosus
- SPECT: single photon emission computed tomography
- STEMI: ST segment elevation myocardial infarction
- SV: stroke volume
- SVT: supraventricular tachycardia
- TAVI: transcatheter aortic valve implantation
- TC: total cholesterol
- TFT: thyroid function test
- TIA: transient ischaemic attack
- TIMI: Thrombolysis In Myocardial Infarction score
- TOE: trans-oesophageal echocardiography
- tPA: tissue plasminogen activator
- TTE: transthoracic echocardiography
- TTP: Thombotic Thrombocytopenic Purpura
- $TXA_2$: thromboxane
- U&E: urea and electrolytes
- UA: unstable angina
- UFH: unfractionated heparin
- VF: ventricular fibrillation
- VSD: ventricular septal defects
- VT: ventricular tachycardia

# An explanation of the text

The book is divided into two parts covering the clinical aspects of cardiology, including investigations and prescribing, and a self-assessment section. We have used bullet points to keep the text concise and supplemented this with a range of diagrams, pictures and MICRO-boxes (explained below).

Where possible we have endeavoured to include treatment options for the conditions covered. Nevertheless, drug sensitivities and clinical practices are constantly under review, so always check your local guidelines for up to date information.

You will find the following resources useful to find out more about any of the drugs mentioned in this book:

- British National Formulary (BNF) (http://www.bnf.org/bnf/index.htm)
- The electronic Medicines Compendium (eMC) (http://www.medicines.org.uk/emc/)

---

**MICRO-facts**

These boxes expand on the text and contain clinically relevant facts and memorable summaries of the essential information.

---

**MICRO-print**

These boxes contain additional information to the text that may interest certain readers but is not essential for everybody to learn.

---

**MICRO-case**

These boxes contain clinical cases relevant to the text and include a number of summary bullet points to highlight the key learning objectives.

---

**MICRO-references**

These boxes contain references to important clinical research and national guidance.

# Part 1

# Cardiology and the cardiovascular system

# 1

# A guide to cardiac history

## 1.1 PRESENTING COMPLAINT

### CHEST PAIN

Site

- Cardiac pain is most commonly central in the chest, retro-sternal or epigastric.
- Pain that is felt in the sides of the chest or well-localized pain is more likely to be mechanical.

Onset

- Sudden (usual) or gradual.
- What was the patient doing when the pain started?

Character

- Crushing, squeezing or a sensation of pressure may represent cardiac ischaemia.
- Severe or 'tearing' pain may be associated with aortic dissection.
- Stabbing pain may be associated with pericarditis or pleurisy.

> ### MICRO-facts
>
> Levine's sign (a clenched fist held over the sternum to describe pain character) is associated with ischaemic pain but has a low positive predictive value. The strongest predictive features of cardiac pain are an association with exercise and radiation to the shoulders or arms. Tenderness in the chest wall does not preclude cardiac chest pain but may be a useful negative predictor.

Radiation

- Radiation to the jaw, arm and hand may occur in ischaemic pain.

### Associated features

- Autonomic symptoms: sweating, clamminess, anxiety, nausea and breathlessness.
- Other cardiac symptoms (see below).

### Timing

- Risk of Acute coronary syndrome (ACS) is threefold higher in the 3 hours after waking.
- Continuous pain over several days is unlikely to be cardiac.

### Exacerbating and alleviating factors

- Relationship to activity, cold temperatures or large meals.
- Relationship to specific movements suggests musculoskeletal pain.
- Alleviating factors: cardiac pain may respond to glyceryl trinitrate (GTN) within minutes; note that oesophageal spasm may also respond to GTN spray but does so much more slowly.
- Pericardial pain is exacerbated by inspiration (like pleuritic chest pain) and may be relieved by sitting upright or leaning forward.

> ### MICRO-facts
> An atypical presentation of myocardial infarction (MI) without pain can occur in elderly patients or those with conditions such as diabetes mellitus and rheumatoid arthritis. Sometimes termed a 'silent' MI.

### BREATHLESSNESS

- Onset, timing and exacerbating factors.
- Associated cough, sputum production or wheeze may suggest a respiratory cause.
- Assess for orthopnoea by asking about the number of pillows the patients needs to sleep and whether they are breathless on lying flat.
- Paroxysmal nocturnal dyspnoea (PND).
- If exercise tolerance is limited by breathlessness, record the current exercise capability and grade it by NYHA class (see Section 5.2, Chronic heart failure).

> ### MICRO-facts
> The absence of both PND and orthopnoea has a strong negative predictive value for the presence of heart failure in those not taking heart failure medication.

- Also record the trend in symptoms, i.e. a rapid deterioration is more concerning than chronically poor exercise tolerance.

## PALPITATIONS

- Onset: gradual or sudden.
- Timing and frequency of episodes: ask about precipitating factors (exercise, stress, caffeine intake, smoking and alcohol) or any techniques used to terminate palpitations.
- Ask the patient to tap out the rhythm to determine regularity.
- Ask about associated pre-syncopal and syncopal symptoms.
- Associated chest pain or breathlessness implies decompensation.

## SYNCOPE

- Describe pre-syncopal symptoms.
- Describe the situation in which syncope occurred, e.g. syncope occurring upon standing up from a recumbent or sitting position implies a postural hypotension.
- Association with palpitations, exercise or recent alterations in drug prescription.
- Association with neck position, e.g. due to vertebrobasilar insufficiency.
- Syncopal symptoms while in the supine position are a worrying feature.

## OTHER SYMPTOMS

- Leg swelling and leg pain:
    - Peripheral oedema may be a result of heart failure.
    - Oedema and pain may be due to deep vein thrombosis related to pulmonary embolism causing non-cardiac chest pain.
    - Pain in the calves on walking that eases with rest is called intermittent claudication and is usually caused by peripheral arterial obstruction.
- Malaise and fatigue may be caused by low cardiac output in heart failure.
- Nausea and anorexia may be caused by hepatic congestion in heart failure.

# 1.2 PAST MEDICAL HISTORY

- Previous occurrence of angina, and if so the frequency and precipitators.
- Previous myocardial infarctions and treatments.
- Previous cardiac investigations such as echocardiograms, perfusion scans and angiograms.
- Previous cardiac intervention such as angioplasty or pacing devices.
- Previous cardiac surgery including coronary bypass surgery and valvular surgery.
- Congenital cardiac conditions.
- History of conditions that are risk factors for ischaemic heart disease such as diabetes, hypertension and hypercholesterolaemia.
- History of conditions that are risk factors for infective endocarditis (e.g. recent dental work, invasive procedures such as colonoscopy, and intravenous drug use).
- History of previous rheumatic fever (may result in valvular disease).

- Recent viral illness if pericarditis or myocarditis is suspected.
- Enquire about conditions such as Marfan's syndrome which may cause aortic root dilatation or aortic dissection.
- A history of stomach ulcers or severe gastritis may require caution in the use of anti-platelet medications, particularly aspirin.

## 1.3 DRUG HISTORY

- Ask about any recent changes to prescriptions, particularly in association with syncopal symptoms or myocarditis as these may be drug induced.
- Ask in particular about current cardiac medications.
- Ask about warfarin use and the latest INR.
- Consider the possible cardio-toxic profile of certain medications:
  - Anti-neoplastic agents, e.g. doxorubicin, cyclophosphamide, paclitaxel
  - Tachycardia-inducing drugs such as salbutamol
  - QTc prolonging medications (see Chapter 12, QTc section)
- Ask about drug allergies and clarify the reaction type.

## 1.4 FAMILY HISTORY

- Enquire about risk factors for ischaemic heart disease: first-degree female relative with a heart attack at less than 65 years of age or a first-degree male relative with a heart attack at less than 55 years of age.
- Enquire about a family history of sudden cardiac death, unexplained death or cardiac defibrillator insertions that may suggest inherited channelopathies such as Brugada syndrome or hypertrophic obstructive cardiomyopathy.
- Enquire about conditions such as familial hypercholesterolaemia or Marfan's syndrome.

## 1.5 SOCIAL HISTORY

- Smoking in pack years (number of cigarettes smoked daily × years smoked/20; e.g. 20 cigarettes per day for 20 years is 20 pack-years).
- Excessive alcohol consumption can cause dilated cardiomyopathy.
- Illicit drug use can cause arrhythmias or cardiomyopathy.
- There is specific guidance relating to driving for patients who have had an ischaemic cardiac event, transient loss of consciousness or cardiac device insertion; this can be found on the UK Driver and Vehicle Licensing Agency (DVLA) website.

> **MICRO-reference**
> The DVLA website has condition-specific guidelines (https://www.gov.uk/health-conditions-and-driving).

# A guide to cardiac examination

## 2.1 GENERAL INSPECTION

- Does the patient appear unwell?
- Does the patient appear breathless or cyanosed: check use of oxygen (type of mask; percentage oxygen), is the patient propped up on pillows?

## 2.2 PERIPHERAL SIGNS OF CARDIOVASCULAR DISEASE

### HANDS

- Colour and temperature.
- Capillary refill time: raise hand to the level of the heart, press for 5 seconds, release and count time to refill.
- Tar staining (from cigarettes).
- Nail clubbing.
- Digital infarcts or nail fold splinters.
- Rare signs of infective endocarditis on the palmar aspect: Janeway lesions and Osler's nodes.

---

### MICRO-facts

Cardiac causes of nail clubbing:
- Cyanotic congenital heart disease
- Infective endocarditis
- Atrial myxoma

---

### FACE

- Cyanosis or pallor under the tongue.
- Poor dentition may provide a source of bacteraemia for infective endocarditis.
- Malar flush may be present in mitral stenosis or pulmonary hypertension.

> ## MICRO-facts
>
> **Hyperlipidaemia:** Xanthelasma, xanthomata (on Achilles tendon) and corneal arcus
>
> **Marfan's syndrome:** Arachnodactyly, tall stature, high arched palate, increased flexibility
>
> **Infective endocarditis:** Osler's nodes, Janeway lesions, splinter haemorrhages, Roth's spots

## PULSES AND BLOOD PRESSURE

### Radial

- Assess rate and rhythm and check for radio-radial and radio-femoral delay.

### Brachial or carotid pulse

*Volume*

- Variation in pulse volume and blood pressure is seen with respiration (increases in expiration and decreases in inspiration due to a rise and fall in intrathoracic pressure, respectively).
- When exaggerated (>10 mmHg change in systolic BP in inspiration), this is known as **pulsus paradoxus** and occurs if intrathoracic pressure decreases in COPD or asthma or when pericardial pathology alters the heart's ability to expand (see Section 7.3).
- **Low volume pulse** is caused by hypovolaemia, peripheral vascular disease or a decreased pulse pressure as happens in mitral and aortic stenosis.
- **High volume pulse** is caused by hypertension, age, exercise, anaemia, $CO_2$ retention or pregnancy.

*Character*

- **Hyperdynamic pulse** is a large-volume bounding pulse seen in anaemia, sepsis, thyrotoxicosis and pregnancy.
- **Slow-rising pulse (pulsus parvus et tardus)** is a pulse increasing gradually in volume that occurs with aortic stenosis.
- **Bisferiens pulse** is a slow-rising pulse with two systolic peaks, felt in aortic stenosis combined with aortic regurgitation.
- **Pulsus alternans** alternates between normal and low volume and occurs in conditions such as mitral or aortic valve stenosis, severe ventricular failure or effusive pericarditis.
- **Collapsing pulse (water hammer)** has an early peak with a rapid decrease in volume that can be exaggerated by raising the arm above the level of the heart (occurs in severe aortic regurgitation).

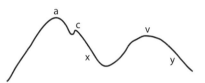

**Figure 2.1** JVP waveform. 'a' wave – right atrial contraction, 'c' wave – tricuspid closure with ventricular contraction, 'x' descent – right atrial relaxation, 'v' wave – right atrial venous filling, 'y' descent – atrial emptying with tricuspid opening.

Jugular Venous Pressure (JVP)

- If visible, the JVP should appear as a diffuse two-peaked pulsation between the two heads of the sternocleidomastoid (see Figure 2.1).
- It alters with inspiration and can be occluded with gentle pressure.
- The height of the JVP above the level of the sternal angle should be measured with the patient reclining at 45 degrees, the usual upper limit of normal height is 3 cm.
- Increased JVP height may reflect increased right atrial pressure:
  - Cor pulmonale
  - Right heart failure as part of congestive cardiac failure
  - Fluid overload

---

**MICRO-print**

Kussmaul's sign – JVP rises in inspiration (seen in impaired right ventricular filling with constrictive pericarditis and pericardial effusion)

Cannon waves – contraction of right atrium against a closed tricuspid valve (seen in complete heart block)

Large 'a' waves – delayed or restricted right ventricular filling (seen in tricuspid stenosis)

Large 'v' waves – tricuspid regurgitation

---

# 2.3 EXAMINATION OF THE PRECORDIUM

## INSPECTION

- Central sternotomy scar
- Lateral surgical scars due to mitral valvotomy
- Evidence of pacing (pacemaker box usually below left clavicle)
- Chest deformity: pectus excavatum, pectus carinatum

Cardiology and the cardiovascular system

## PALPATION

- Assess for deviation of the apex beat, which is usually located at the fifth intercostal space in the mid-clavicular line.
- Palpate the chest for heaves parasternally (right ventricular hypertrophy), heaves at the apex (left ventricular hypertrophy) and thrills (palpable murmurs).

## AUSCULTATION

- First heart sound (S1): closure of the mitral and tricuspid valves
- Second heart sound (S2): closure of the aortic and pulmonary valves (this is physiologically split on inspiration)

### Additional sounds

- A third heart sound (S3) is heard early in diastole – it is pathological in patients above 40 years of age when it is most likely to be associated with reduced left ventricular function or mitral regurgitation.
- A fourth heart sound (S4) precedes S1 – it is always pathological and caused by atrial contraction against the non-complant left ventricle.
- Pericardial rub is a harsh sound heard in pericarditis – characteristically scratchy and heard both in systole and diastole.

> ## MICRO-facts
>
> An onomatopoeic memory aid for recognizing the third heart sound is to remember the word 'kentucky' where S1 = ken, S2 = tuck, S3 = y. Similarly, the word 'tennessee' may help to remember that the S4 sound appears before S1, where S4 = ten, S1 = nes, S2 = see.

### Volume change

- Systemic and pulmonary hypertension increase the volume of the aortic and pulmonary heart S2 sounds, respectively (often termed a loud A2 and a loud P2, respectively).
- A calcific or immobile valve may shut quietly or silently, while a click may be heard with a mobile valve leaflet.
- Quiet heart sounds may occur in the presence of a reduced cardiac output, pericardial effusion or emphysema.

### Splitting of heart sounds

- Delay in right ventricular emptying causes exaggerated S2 splitting.
- Delay in left ventricular emptying reverses the splitting of S2 so splitting occurs in expiration.
- Reverse splitting (A2 after P2) occurs in left bundle branch block.
- Fixed splitting is seen with atrial septal defect.

> **MICRO-print**
> **Left-sided murmurs** are accentuated on expiration, as increased thoracic pressure increases cardiac output from the left ventricle.
>
> **Right-sided murmurs** are accentuated on inspiration as a negative thoracic pressure increases the blood flow through the right-sided cardiac chambers.

Murmurs
- A murmur is caused by turbulent blood flow, usually through an abnormal valve.
- A **flow murmur** can develop across a normal valve when the blood flow velocity is abnormally increased as in high cardiac output states, e.g. thyrotoxicosis, anaemia, sepsis and pregnancy.
- Describe a murmur according to:
  - Timing: systolic, diastolic or continuous (note that a systolic murmur is simultaneous with the carotid pulsation)
  - Location on the precordium
  - Volume (1–6) may not be related to valve disease severity as murmurs may become quieter with increasing severity
  - Quality: high pitched, blowing
  - Radiation
  - Any additional sounds

# 2.4 COMPLETING THE CARDIAC EXAMINATION

- Auscultate the lung bases and palpate the sacrum and ankles for signs of dependent pitting oedema.
- Palpate the liver to assess for congestion or pulsatility.
- Assess for splenomegaly that may be present in infective endocarditis.
- Perform fundoscopy for signs of hypertensive retinopathy or Roth's spots that may be seen in infective endocarditis.
- Perform a urine dipstick test for haematuria that may be present in infective endocarditis.

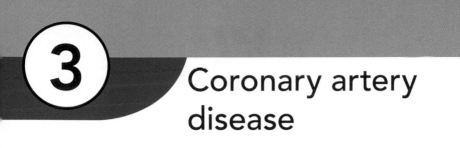

# 3 Coronary artery disease

*Symptoms characterized by reduced blood flow to the myocardium*

> **MICRO-print**
> The latest national public statistics for coronary artery disease (CAD) (British Heart Foundation, UK, and Centers for Disease Control and Prevention, USA) indicate that:
> - CAD is the leading single cause of death in the UK and the USA.
> - CAD causes approximately 25% of deaths in the USA (2009), and 12–17% of deaths in the UK (2010).
> - 124,000 heart attacks occur annually in the UK.
> - 1998–2008 saw a 49% decrease in deaths in males aged 55–64 in the UK.
> - £3.2 billion was spent on CAD in the UK in 2006.

## 3.1 ANATOMY OF THE CORONARY ARTERIES

The coronary arteries run in the subepicardial connective tissue (see Figure 3.1).

- **Right coronary artery** (RCA) arises from the anterior sinus behind the aortic cusp and:
  - Runs between the pulmonary trunk and the right atrium
  - Continues posteriorly along the atrioventricular groove to give off branches:
    - **Marginal** branch runs along the lower costal surface to reach the apex.
    - **Posterior descending interventricular branch** runs towards the apex of the heart in the posterior interventricular groove.
- **Left coronary artery** arises from the posterior sinus behind the aortic cusp and:
  - As the left main stem between the pulmonary trunk and the left atrium
  - Enters the atrioventricular groove and divides into:
    - **Anterior descending interventricular** branch runs towards the apex in the anterior interventricular groove and gives off diagonal and septal branches.
    - **Circumflex** branch winds around to the back of the heart in the atrioventricular groove and gives off the left marginal branch(es).

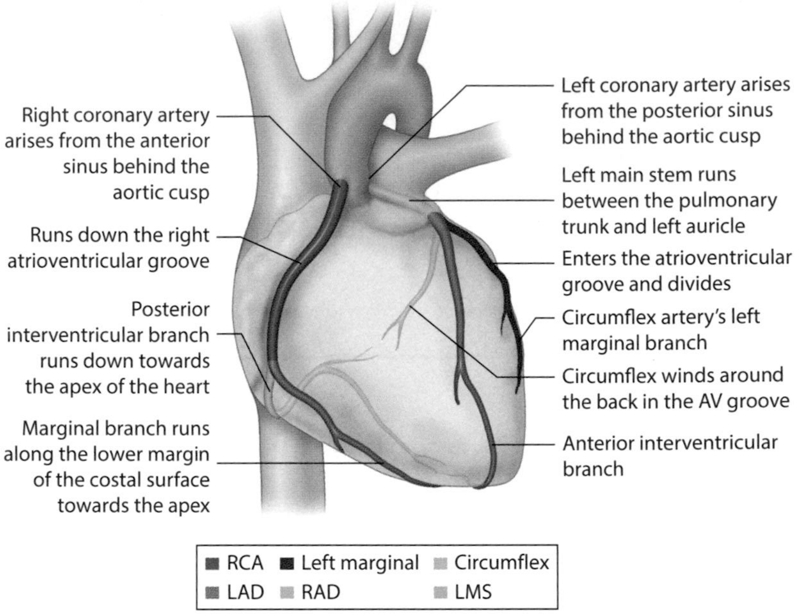

Right coronary artery arises from the anterior sinus behind the aortic cusp

Runs down the right atrioventricular groove

Posterior interventricular branch runs down towards the apex of the heart

Marginal branch runs along the lower margin of the costal surface towards the apex

Left coronary artery arises from the posterior sinus behind the aortic cusp

Left main stem runs between the pulmonary trunk and left auricle

Enters the atrioventricular groove and divides

Circumflex artery's left marginal branch

Circumflex winds around the back in the AV groove

Anterior interventricular branch

■ RCA ■ Left marginal ▨ Circumflex
■ LAD ▨ RAD ▨ LMS

**Figure 3.1** Anatomy of the coronary arteries.

| RIGHT CORONARY ARTERY SUPPLIES | LEFT CORONARY ARTERY SUPPLIES |
|---|---|
| RV and RA | LV and LA |
| Part of LA and diaphragmatic surface of LV | |
| Posterior 1/3 of the ventricular septum | Anterior 2/3 of the ventricular septum |
| Sinoatrial node in 65% of the population | Sinoatrial node in 35% of the population |
| Atrioventricular node in 90% of the population | Atrioventricular node in 10% of the population |
| Some of the left bundle branch | Right bundle branch and left bundle branch |

## 3.2 PATHOLOGY OF CAD: ATHEROSCLEROSIS

Coronary arteries:
- Tunica adventitia: outermost layer
- Tunica media: muscular middle layer
- Tunica intima: endothelial inner lining

## ATHEROSCLEROSIS

Early lesion: fatty streak

- Early precursor of the atherosclerotic plaque.
- Present from childhood in the aorta, from adolescence in the coronary arteries.
- Deposition of foam cells in the intima of muscular artery walls:
  - Foam cells are macrophages that migrate into the intima in response to inflammation caused by harmful oxidized low-density lipoprotein (LDL) molecules in the arterial wall.
  - Macrophages ingest lipids through special scavenger receptors.
  - Macrophages may undergo necrosis and rupture, depositing lipids.
- Not all fatty streaks will progress to become atherosclerotic plaques.

Advanced lesion: atherosclerotic plaque

- Two components (see Figure 3.2):
  - *Atheroma:* soft inner core composed of lipids and a periphery of necrotic foam cells and cholesterol crystals – **highly thrombogenic in nature**.
  - *Fibrous capsule:* outer layer composed of smooth muscle cells that have migrated from the media into the intima sequestering the lipid core – **may start to calcify**.
- Plaques become problematic:
  - In angina, increased luminal obstruction will result in a mismatch between $O_2$ delivery in situations of increased demand such as during exercise (usually the stenosis has to be >50% of the arterial lumen diameter [75% cross-sectional area] for symptoms to appear).
  - In acute myocardial infarction, the fibrous capsule erodes or ruptures, exposing the lipid core to the blood and resulting in thrombus formation and distal embolization.

Vulnerable atherosclerotic plaques

- These features make plaques prone to rupture or erosion:
  - **Large-volume, necrotic lipid core**

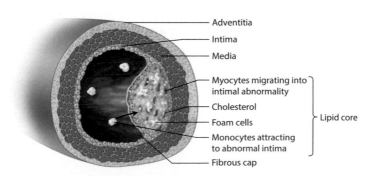

**Figure 3.2** Atherosclerotic plaque components.

Adventitia
Intima
Media
Myocytes migrating into intimal abnormality
Cholesterol
Foam cells
Monocytes attracting to abnormal intima
Fibrous cap
Lipid core

Cardiology and the cardiovascular system

- **Thin fibrous cap**
  - Angiogenesis with haemorrhage within the plaque
  - Release of extracellular proteases by macrophages
  - Inflammation within a thin fibrous cap
- Vulnerable plaque rupture or erosion may be precipitated by high blood pressure and tachycardia due to the changes in shear stress over the plaque.

## MICRO-facts

Plaque rupture or erosion may be independent of plaque size and luminal stenosis, hence may not be preceded by stable angina.

## RISK FACTORS FOR CAD

Risk factors predisposing to coronary artery disease may:
- Be modifiable or non-modifiable
- Encourage formation of unstable atherosclerotic plaques
- Precipitate plaque rupture or erosion and subsequent thrombosis

### MICRO-print
Acute myocardial infarctions occur most commonly in the morning. This may be due to a morning increase in blood pressure and vasoconstriction secondary to a heightened sympathetic drive (precipitants of plaque rupture or erosion) and also due to increased platelet aggregation in the morning (propagation of thrombus formation).

| NON-MODIFIABLE RISK FACTORS | |
|---|---|
| Age | Atherosclerotic lesions mature with age. Declining testosterone levels and oestrogen levels in ageing men and women, respectively, result in a loss of their cardioprotective effect |
| Male gender | Oestrogens have a protective effect in pre-menopausal women. Effects of individual risk factors also differ between gender and may confer protection to women |
| Family history | First-degree relative with stroke or CAD <65 years (♀) or <55 years (♂) |

*Continued*

| MODIFIABLE RISK FACTORS AND RELATIVE RISK RATIOS | | |
|---|---|---|
| | RR (♂–♀)[a] | |
| Diabetes mellitus | 1.69–2.74 | Risk of a patient with diabetes having a first myocardial infarction is approximately that of a non-diabetic patient who has already had a myocardial infarction |
| Hypertension | 1.46–1.42 | Enhances the atherosclerotic process Contributes to plaque instability and rupture Causes left ventricular hypertrophy increasing myocardial $O_2$ demand and decreasing coronary artery reserve |
| Smoking | 1.41–1.42 | Smoking increases inflammation in atherosclerosis Smoking affects high-density lipoprotein (HDL) levels and fibrinogen levels A single cigarette increases platelet aggregation and the risk of plaque rupture and thrombus formation Risk returns to that of a non-smoker after 10 years of cessation at any age |
| Physical inactivity | 1.28–1.36 | Inactivity increases the risk of obesity Exercise decreases the basal heart rate (basal rate >70 beats per minute is associated with a higher risk of CAD) |
| Hypercholesterolaemia | 1.22–1.23 | Plaques with a large lipid core are unstable Elevated LDL and low HDL levels increase risk Total cholesterol to HDL ratio is a useful clinical measure |
| Obesity | 1.20–1.19 | Waist circumference may be a better indicator than body mass index |
| Triglycerides | 1.06–1.33 | Risk factor independent of total cholesterol levels Increases risk of CAD more significantly in women |

*Continued*

Cardiology and the cardiovascular system

| NOVEL RISK FACTORS | |
|---|---|
| Chronic inflammation | Rheumatoid arthritis may lead to at least a twofold increase in risk of myocardial infarction and stroke |
| Type A personality | |
| High C-reactive protein | |
| High fibrinogen levels | |
| High homocysteine levels | |
| Abnormal ankle brachial index | |
| Low income | |
| Ethnic group, e.g. South Asians | |
| Small and dense LDL particle | |

[a] Interheart study: Schnohr P, Jensen JS, Scharling H, et al. Coronary heart disease risk factors ranked by importance for the individual and community. *European Heart Journal* 2002; 23: 620–626.
Definition of relative risk (RR): chance of an event occurring in a population exposed to a factor compared to the chance of the event occurring in an unexposed population.

Metabolic syndrome

- A collection of factors closely linked with obesity that increase the risk of CAD, certain cancers, hypotestosteronemia in men and non-alcoholic fatty liver disease.
- It is diagnosed when at least three of the five criteria are met (International Diabetes Federation and American Heart Association Criteria):

| Abdominal obesity (waist circumference) | |
|---|---|
| Men | >102 cm (>40 in) |
| Women | >88 cm (>35 in) |
| Asian men | >90 cm (>35 in) |
| Asian women | >80 cm (>32 in) |
| Triglycerides | ≥1.7 mmol/L or on therapy |
| HDL cholesterol | |
| Men | <1.03 mmol/L or on therapy |
| Women | <1.29 mmol/L or on therapy |
| Blood pressure | ≥130/≥85 mmHg or on therapy |
| Fasting plasma glucose | ≥5.6 mmol/L or on therapy |

MICRO-reference
International Diabetes Federation website on the metabolic syndrome:
http://www.idf.org/metabolic-syndrome

## 3.3 PRIMARY PREVENTION

- Mortality from coronary heart disease has almost halved in the last three decades:
    - Half of this decrease is attributed to better treatment measures, such as the use of anti-hypertensives, statins, aspirin and interventions like primary angioplasty.
    - The remainder of the decrease is attributable to modification of risk factors.
- **Primary prevention** modifies risk factors in individuals with no clinical evidence of CAD, e.g. anti-hypertensives, diabetes management, smoking cessation.
- **Secondary prevention** aims to reduce recurrence of events and improves survival in those who have had a cardiovascular event, e.g. aspirin use in patients with angina, angiotensin-converting enzyme inhibitors post-MI.

## MICRO-facts

**'Good cholesterol versus bad cholesterol'**
Apolipoproteins are proteins that bind lipids.
**Apolipoprotein B makes up low-density lipoprotein (LDL, 'bad cholesterol')**

- LDL invades the arterial wall, is oxidized and results in inflammation attracting macrophages that engulf the LDL and become foam cells.
- Familial hypercholesterolaemia is autosomal dominant and associated with high levels of LDL and CAD risk.

**Apolipoprotein A1 makes up high-density lipoprotein (HDL, 'good cholesterol')**

- HDL composed of apolipoprotein A1 undertakes reverse cholesterol transport from foam macrophages in the arteries to the liver and faeces.

- **Tertiary prevention** aims to prevent complications, e.g. closure of post-infarction ventricular septal defects.

Cardiology and the cardiovascular system

## CARDIOVASCULAR RISK PREDICTION CHARTS

- To implement primary prevention, primary care providers can use the World Health Organization cardiovascular disease risk prediction charts; these are tailored to geographical subregions.
- These predict the risk of developing a cardiovascular event in the next 10 years (includes cardiovascular death, new-onset angina, myocardial infarction, transient ischaemic attacks and stroke) (see Figure 3.3).
- Risk factors taken into account:
  - Gender
  - Age (useful for individuals up to 70 years of age)
  - Smoking status (cessation in the past 5 years is still classified as 'smoker')
  - Systolic blood pressure
  - Serum total cholesterol: HDL ratio

Charts can help physicians make decisions on the provision of treatment for:

- Hypertension (treatment recommended at CAD risk >20% if ambulatory blood pressure or home blood pressure >135/85 mmHg) (see Section 10.5).
- Hyperlipidaemia (CAD risk >10% over the next 10 years warrants the use of statins).
- In some cases, these will be elevated enough in themselves to warrant treatment.
- Implement lifestyle changes and medications.
- Do not use the chart for treatment decisions in:

| CLINICALLY ESTABLISHED CVD | SECONDARY PREVENTION IMPLEMENTED |
|---|---|
| Diabetes mellitus type 1 or 2 | Treat appropriately and implement primary prevention |
| Renal dysfunction | Treat appropriately and implement primary prevention |
| Familial hyperlipidaemia Total cholesterol: HDL >6 | Statin therapy |
| Persistently raised BP >160/100 mmHg Hypertension with end-organ damage | Treat blood pressure using guidelines |

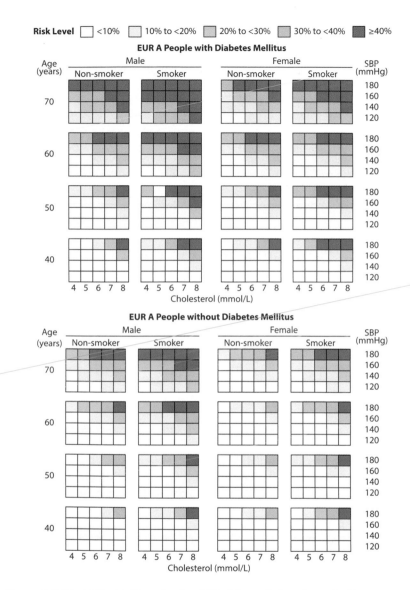

**Figure 3.3** World Health Organization CAD risk prediction charts for Europe subregion A including the United Kingdom.

## MICRO-facts

In addition to decreasing plasma LDL and plaque lipid content and thrombogenicity, statins have an anti-inflammatory action and increase collagen:inflammatory cell ratio in plaques, making them less vulnerable. Some indications for the use of statins include the following:

- Primary prevention of CAD if 10-year risk is >10% or TC:HDL >6
- Secondary prevention of CAD
- Familial hyperlipidaemia
- Diabetes mellitus in patients >40 years or younger if target end-organ damage or multiple risk factors are present

## 3.4 PRESENTATIONS AND PATHOPHYSIOLOGY OF CAD

- Mismatch between myocardial $O_2$ requirement and supply manifests as ischaemic chest pain:
  - Stable chronic angina
  - Acute coronary syndrome (ACS): acute myocardial ischaemia
    - Unstable angina (UA)
    - Non-ST segment elevation myocardial infarction (NSTEMI)
    - ST segment elevation myocardial infarction (STEMI)
- The diagnostic triad in ACS consists of history, ECG changes and cardiac enzymes.
- Chest pain at rest or minimal exertion suggests ACS rather than chronic stable angina.
- Elevated cardiac markers will differentiate between UA and NSTEMI/STEMI.
- ST segment elevation will differentiate between NSTEMI and STEMI.
- The table below outlines the pathophysiology underlying stable angina and ACS.

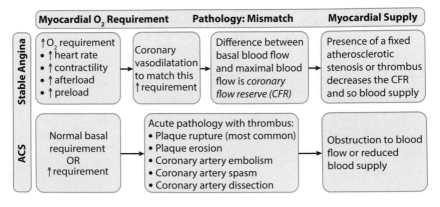

| | Myocardial $O_2$ Requirement | Pathology: Mismatch | | Myocardial Supply |
|---|---|---|---|---|
| **Stable Angina** | ↑$O_2$ requirement • ↑ heart rate • ↑ contractility • ↑ afterload • ↑ preload | Coronary vasodilatation to match this ↑requirement | Difference between basal blood flow and maximal blood flow is *coronary flow reserve (CFR)* | Presence of a fixed atherosclerotic stenosis or thrombus decreases the CFR and so blood supply |
| **ACS** | Normal basal requirement OR ↑requirement | | Acute pathology with thrombus: • Plaque rupture (most common) • Plaque erosion • Coronary artery embolism • Coronary artery spasm • Coronary artery dissection | Obstruction to blood flow or reduced blood supply |

**Differences between the various CAD presentations**

| PRESENTATION | PATHOPHYSIOLOGICAL | DIAGNOSTIC | | |
| --- | --- | --- | --- | --- |
| | | HISTORY | ECG CHANGES | CARDIAC MARKERS |
| Chronic stable angina | Fixed stenosis >50% and decreased coronary reserve flow | Chest pain on exertion <10 minutes | Normal at Rest ST depression or T inversion on exertion | ↔ |
| Unstable angina | Acute thrombus formation and resolution OR Severe stenoses >90% interfering with basal coronary blood supply | Chest pain at rest or minimal exertion | ST depression or T inversion at rest May be normal | ↔ |
| NSTEMI | Acute thrombus Partial occlusion | Chest pain >20 minutes | ST depression or T inversion at rest May be normal | ↑ |
| STEMI | Acute thrombus Complete occlusion | Chest pain >20 minutes | ST elevation at rest | ↑ |

## CHRONIC STABLE ANGINA

> ### MICRO-facts
>
> The leading cause of angina is CAD but any factor decreasing myocardial $O_2$ supply will result in angina.
> - Coronary vasospasm → Prinzmetal's angina
> - Short diastole decreasing coronary filling:
>   - Tachyarrhythmias
>   - Aortic stenosis
>   - Hypertrophic obstructive cardiomyopathy
> - Decreased $O_2$ provision → severe anaemia or hypoxia

- Stable angina is a result of inadequate myocardial $O_2$ provision in states of increased $O_2$ utilization within the context of a fixed reduction in coronary reserve flow.
- It precipitates chest pain on physical exertion, with severe emotion or in cold air.
- Typical anginal pain has all the following features:
  - Central chest pain, constricting in nature
  - Precipitated by exertion
  - Relieved by rest or glyceryl trinitrate (GTN) in about 5 minutes
    - Two of the above features: atypical angina
    - One or no features: non-anginal chest pain

### INVESTIGATIONS

| Laboratory tests | FBC | Severe anaemia may cause angina |
|---|---|---|
| | U&E | Look for renal dysfunction |
| | Fasting lipids | Dyslipidaemia as a risk factor for CAD |
| | Glucose | Diabetes as a risk factor for CAD |
| | Thyroid function | Thyrotoxicosis and hypothyroidism may present with angina |
| **ECG** | Resting | Look for resting changes indicative of ischaemia, tachyarrhythmias or previous MI |
| | Exercise | Look for changes of ischaemia (see Chapter 12) |

**Further tests: guidelines for the diagnosis of CAD in suspected stable angina** (see NICE guidelines 2010; see Chapter 16 for details of these investigations). Risk stratify patients according to typicality of chest pain, risk factors, age and gender:
- <10% probability of CAD: seek other possible causes for the chest pain.
- 10–29% probability of CAD: should be offered CT calcium scoring.

- 30–60% probability of CAD: should be offered non-invasive functional testing, e.g. myocardial perfusion scan or stress echocardiogram.
- 61–90% probability of CAD: should be offered invasive angiography.
- >90% probability of CAD: should be started on treatment for stable angina.

---

**MICRO-print**

Cardiac syndrome X is the combination of chest pain and cardiac ischaemia suggested by stress tests and ECG findings. However, these patients have a normal coronary angiography. Prinzmetal's angina should be excluded. Symptomatic treatment may be continued.

---

**MICRO-reference**

National Institute for Health and Care Excellence. Chest pain of recent onset: assessment and diagnosis of recent onset chest pain or discomfort of suspected cardiac origin. NICE guidelines [CG95]. London: National Institute for Health and Care Excellence, 2010. http://www.nice.org.uk/guidance/cg95/chapter/guidance

---

**ECG changes in acute MI**

ECG changes in ischaemia are:

- T wave inversion, ST segment depression (seen co-incident with chest pain)

ECG changes in an acute STEMI classically appear in the following chronological order:

- Giant, peaked, hyperacute T waves
- ST segment elevation (>2 mm in chest leads or >1 mm in limb leads)
- Pathological Q waves (>25% height of R wave, >0.04 seconds wide, inverted T waves)
- Return of ST segment to normal and inversion of T wave with persisting ischaemia over about 48 hours

STEMI can present with left bundle branch block (LBBB) indicating wide anterior wall necrosis.

In an acute posterior STEMI, ST segment depression is seen in the V1–V3, diagnosis assisted by the use of posterior chest ECG leads.

Note that ST segment elevation does not always indicate STEMI, differentials include:

- Myocarditis
- Acute myo-pericarditis (saddle-shaped ST segment elevation)
- Ventricular aneurysm (persistent ST segment elevation)

Cardiology and the cardiovascular system

Localizing an infarct

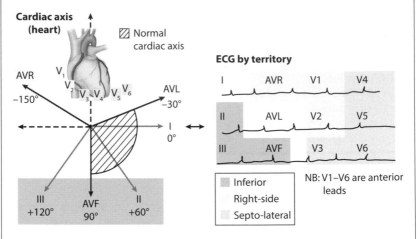

Figure 3.4 Cardiac axis and placement of chest leads.

| REGION | LEADS | ARTERIAL OCCLUSION |
|---|---|---|
| Anterior | V1–V3 | LAD artery |
| Antero-septal | V1–V4 | LAD artery |
| Inferior | II, III, aVF | RCA |
| Lateral | I, aVL, V5–V6 | Circumflex artery and diagonal branch of LAD |
| Right | V4R–V6R aVR | RCA |
| Posterior | V1–V3 | PDA and circumflex artery |

In a STEMI, look for

- ST segment elevation in a region (see Figure 3.4)
- Reciprocal ischaemic changes in the other regions (ST segment depression and T wave inversion)

## MANAGEMENT

Adopt a five-step approach to management of chronic stable angina:

1. **Communicate** with the patient:
   a. New-onset chest pain suggestive of angina should trigger a cardiology referral or rapid access chest pain clinic referral.
2. **Relieve symptoms** with GTN spray.

3. **Prevent symptoms** with anti-anginal therapy (see Section 17.1 for anti-anginal mechanism):

| NICE GUIDELINES ON ANGINA MANAGEMENT, 2011 | |
|---|---|
| 1st line | Beta-blocker or calcium channel blocker (depending on contraindications) |
| 2nd line | Beta-blocker + calcium channel blocker |
| 3rd line | Consider adding a long-acting nitrate, ivabradine, nicorandil or ranolazine |

4. **Secondary prevention** by addressing risk factors using ABCDE:
   **A**spirin 75 mg once daily, **A**CE inhibitors
   **B**lood pressure control
   **C**holesterol control (statins)
   **D**iabetes control
   **E**xercise, smoking cessation and diet
5. **Consider revascularization** if lack of symptomatic control:
   a. Percutaneous coronary intervention (PCI)
   b. Coronary artery bypass graft (CABG)

> # MICRO-facts
> If a patient develops chest pain, which persists after 10 minutes and two doses of GTN, then call an ambulance.

## ACUTE CORONARY SYNDROME

### SYMPTOMS

- Central, crushing dull chest pain radiating to either arm, neck or jaw
- Appearing at rest or on exertion and persisting >20 minutes and unrelieved by GTN spray
- Sweating
- Nausea and vomiting
- Shortness of breath

### SIGNS

- Levine's sign: patient describes pain by holding a clenched fist over chest area (unreliable).
- Dyspnoea, diaphoresis and tachycardia.
- Check for signs suggestive of complications such as acute valvular regurgitation or acute ventricular septal defect (heart murmurs), acute heart failure (added heart sounds, raised JVP, bibasal lung crackles) or other tachyarrhythmias (e.g. atrial fibrillation).

INVESTIGATIONS

| Laboratory tests | Cardiac markers | Troponin I or T |
|---|---|---|
| | FBC | Look for anaemia or infection |
| | U&E | Look for renal dysfunction as it affects some drug dosing |
| | Fasting lipids | Obtain a baseline measure of lipid levels within 24 hours<br>May remain artificially low for 8 weeks after event |
| | Glucose | May be elevated due to an acute stress response<br>In diabetics, MI can precipitate diabetic ketoacidosis |
| | D-Dimer | Consider to exclude a pulmonary embolus (PE) if diagnosis unclear |
| | LFT, amylase | Cholecystitis or pancreatitis may present with chest pain |
| **ECG** | Resting (see Chapter 12) | |
| **CXR** | Pulmonary oedema with acute heart failure post-MI<br>Alternative diagnosis (pneumothorax, widened mediastinum in aortic dissection) | |
| **ABG** | Not routine, look for hypoxia due to dyspnoea or alternative diagnosis (pneumothorax, PE) | |
| **2D Echo** | Wall motion abnormalities are suggestive of ischaemia or infarction | |

---

**Initial management for all patients with ACS**

1. **ABC** approach: environment with resuscitation facilities and continuous monitoring
2. **High flow O$_2$** 15 L/min through a non-rebreathe mask if patient is hypoxic (caution should be exercised in the prolonged use of high-flow O$_2$ in patients with chronic obstructive pulmonary disease)
3. **ECG** trace and immediate interpretation
4. **Secure IV access** and obtain initial blood investigations including cardiac enzymes
5. **Drug** treatment
   a. Aspirin 300 mg orally
   b. GTN spray sublingually to relieve pain
   c. Diamorphine 2.5–10 mg intravenously (IV) to relieve pain and anxiety + metoclopramide 10 mg IV

# MICRO-facts

**Troponins I and T are parts of regulatory proteins in skeletal and cardiac muscle.** Assays can detect the subtypes specific to cardiac muscle in myocardial injury, yielding high sensitivity and specificity (see Figure 3.5).

- Best measured serially to demonstrate a rise.
- Rise as early as 3 hours, peak between 12 and 24 hours.
- Single best measure at 12 hours since chest pain.
- Newer high sensitivity troponin assays can exclude ACS at 6 hours after onset of symptoms.
- Remain elevated for up to a couple of weeks.
- Use of troponin I or T +/− high sensitivity testing varies by local protocol – consult local guidelines.
- False positives include sepsis, PE, renal failure, cardiac failure, myocarditis and pericarditis.
- Raised troponins have a poorer prognostic value.
- Creatine Kinase-MB (creatine phosphokinase MB) has been replaced by troponins. It peaks at 24 hours and falls to normal within a few days. It is more specific to the myocardium compared with CK (creatine kinase) that is elevated in skeletal muscle trauma, convulsions, surgery or PE.
- More non-specific markers include AST and LDH.

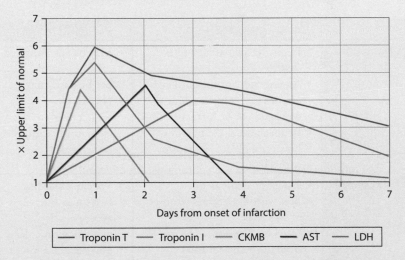

Figure 3.5 Cardiac enzyme release after myocardial infarction. (From bpac[nz]. *The role of troponin testing in primary care.* Best Tests 2009. Available at www.bpac.org.nz.)

> **MICRO-print**
>
> ACS can precipitate endocrine emergencies such as thyrotoxicosis, myxoedema crisis, Addisonian crisis and diabetic ketoacidosis.
> Make sure to record an ECG in patients (of appropriate age and with coronary artery disease risk factors) presenting with these conditions.

## STEMI

1. *Immediate management*

   **Aspirin 300 mg + clopidogrel 300 mg + GTN + opiate pain relief**
   - There are $P2Y_{12}$ receptor antagonists other than clopidogrel, including ticagrelor.

2. *Reperfusion therapy:* **primary PCI** or **thrombolysis**
   - Primary PCI reduces mortality compared to thrombolysis in patients with STEMI and should always be the first choice treatment.
   - However, if the door-to-balloon (primary PCI) time exceeds the door-to-needle (thrombolysis) time by 120 minutes, this benefit is lost.
   - Delayed surgery may be necessary (4–6 weeks) for complications including:
     - Papillary muscle rupture
     - Septal rupture
   - See Section 17.4 for types of intravenous agents used for thrombolysis.

|  | PRIMARY PCI | THROMBOLYSIS |
|---|---|---|
| Advantages | • High arterial patency rates – 90%<br>• Angiography of the coronary arteries can guide medical management or further CABG<br>• Better residual LV function<br>• Low rates of late restenosis with DES | • May be administered early as part of pre-hospital care<br>• No need for catheterization laboratory facilities<br>• Lesser staff requirement |
| Disadvantages | • Operator-dependent<br>• Best within 12 hours of onset of STEMI<br>• Need for a catheterization laboratory and on-call specialized staff<br>• Risks of invasive therapy<br>• Reperfusion arrhythmias commoner | • Systemic bleeding<br>• Risks may outweigh benefits with increasing time delay<br>• Low recanalization rates (60%)<br>• Contraindications exclude up to 10% of patients |

Cardiology and the cardiovascular system

3. *Further medical management*

| Beta-blockers | • Reduce myocardial $O_2$ consumption by lowering HR, BP and contractility.<br>• Limit infarct extent, reduce mortality and incidence of tachyarrhythmias.<br>• Contraindicated in unstable heart failure, bradycardia and hypotension.<br>• Use short-acting agents initially such as metoprolol.<br>• Start at a low dose when the patient is haemodynamically stable. |
|---|---|
| Statins | • High-dose early use reduces mortality (atorvastatin 80 mg PROVE-IT, MIRACL trials) – only in NSTEMI not STEMI.<br>• Higher doses associated with greater side effect profile. |
| Angiotensin-converting enzyme inhibitor (ACEi) | • Start low dose after reperfusion therapy at 24–48 hours when haemodynamically stable.<br>• Especially benefits elderly patients and those with anterior STEMI, high-risk STEMI, previous MI or tachycardia at presentation. |

4. *Late risk stratification and further assessment*
- Monitor all patients for complications post-STEMI or due to reperfusion therapy.
- Routine angiography is not indicated in patients after completed STEMI unless there is ongoing ischaemic chest pain.
  **Assessment for defibrillator implantation**
- Patients who have undergone primary PCI may be considered for defibrillator implantation +/– inpatient electrophysiological studies if:
  - Sustained or pulseless VT/VF post-procedure
  - Non-sustained VT with LV ejection fraction <40% (despite full medical therapy with beta-blocker and angiotensin-converting enzyme inhibitor [ACEi]) post-procedure

## UA/NSTEMI

- Although it is easy to differentiate early between UA/NSTEMI and STEMI by ST segment deviation on ECG, differentiation between UA and NSTEMI is delayed until cardiac enzymes (rapid increase followed by a slow decrease) confirm myocardial damage (NSTEMI).
- The following may be presentations of UA/NSTEMI:
  - Angina at rest
  - Crescendo angina (worsening severity, frequency, duration)
  - New-onset angina

Principles of acute management:
- Emergency management and administration of drugs.
- Risk stratification with an appropriate tool with a view to early reperfusion therapy (evidence shows benefit of early invasive strategy is limited to higher risk groups).
- Late risk stratification of patients on early conservative management with further tests (with a view to late reperfusion therapy).
- Anti-coagulation

1. *Medical management*

| ASPIRIN 300 mg + GTN + OPIATE PAIN RELIEF | |
|---|---|
| **Beta-blockers** | Reduce myocardial $O_2$ consumption by lowering HR, BP and contractility<br>Reduce mortality and incidence of tachyarrhythmias<br>Contraindicated in unstable heart failure, bradycardia and hypotension<br>Use short-acting agents such as metoprolol |
| **Statins** | High-dose early use reduces mortality (atorvastatin 80 mg) |
| **Calcium antagonists** | May help symptomatically but there is no effect on mortality |

2. *Further management*

**Stratify patients** by mortality risk to decide on early invasive or conservative management.
- Examples of risk stratification tools include:
  - TIMI risk score: 14-day mortality risk
  - GRACE score: 6-month mortality risk or in-hospital mortality

| | TIMI (THROMBOLYSIS IN MYOCARDIAL INFARCTION) FACTORS (SCORE OUT OF 7) | GRACE (GLOBAL REGISTRY FOR ACUTE CORONARY EVENTS) FACTORS |
|---|---|---|
| History | Age ≥65 years<br>Aspirin used in the past 7 days<br>≥3 risk factors for CAD | Age |
| Presentation | Coronary stenosis ≥50%<br>2 Angina episodes in past 24 hours | Cardiac arrest, HR, SBP<br>Serum creatinine<br>Congestive heart failure |

*Continued*

| | TIMI (THROMBOLYSIS IN MYOCARDIAL INFARCTION) FACTORS (SCORE OUT OF 7) | GRACE (GLOBAL REGISTRY FOR ACUTE CORONARY EVENTS) FACTORS |
|---|---|---|
| ECG | ST segment deviation | ST segment deviation |
| Enzymes | Elevated cardiac enzymes | Elevated cardiac enzymes (used for in-hospital mortality calculation only) |
| Risk classification | 14-Day mortality risk Score 0–1: 4.7% risk Score 2: 8.3% risk Score 3: 13.2% risk Score 4: 19.9% risk Score 5: 26.2% risk Score 6: 40.9% risk Score 7: 40.9% risk | 6-Month mortality risk Lowest: ≤1.5% risk Low: >1.5–3.0% risk Intermediate: >3.0–6.0% risk High: >6.0–9.0% risk Highest: >9.0% risk |

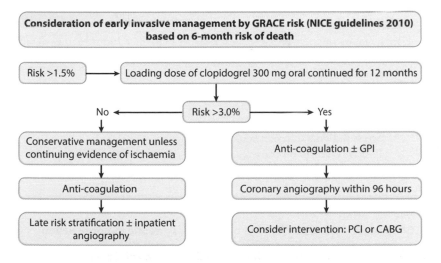

**Consideration of early invasive management by GRACE risk (NICE guidelines 2010) based on 6-month risk of death**

Risk >1.5% → Loading dose of clopidogrel 300 mg oral continued for 12 months

No ← Risk >3.0% → Yes

Conservative management unless continuing evidence of ischaemia

Anti-coagulation ± GPI

Anti-coagulation

Coronary angiography within 96 hours

Late risk stratification ± inpatient angiography

Consider intervention: PCI or CABG

### Early reperfusion therapy for moderate- to high-risk patients

- Management strategy is early angiography with a view to PCI for moderate- to high-risk patients identified using TIMI or GRACE scores.
- Additionally the European Society of Cardiology (ESC) recommends early invasive management in the following situations:
  - Haemodynamic instability
  - Major arrhythmias
  - Diabetes mellitus

Cardiology and the cardiovascular system

**Anti-coagulation** (see Section 17.4)

- Fondaparinux if PCI/CABG not planned within 24 hours and renal function adequate (also offer unfractionated heparin [UFH] during PCI to these patients).
- Consider UFH if PCI or CABG planned within 24 hours or in patients with renal impairment.
- Bivalirudin as an alternative to heparin for angiography planned within 24 hours for patients not already on a glycoprotein inhibitor or fondaparinux.

**Glycoprotein IIb/IIIa inhibitors (GPI)** (see Section 17.5)

- Abciximab can be used as an adjunct to PCI in high-risk cases.
- Eptifibatide or tirofiban in high-risk cases if angiography planned within the next 96 hours.

### Late risk stratification for patients with early conservative management

- Risk stratification assesses the benefit of late invasive imaging and reperfusion therapy.
- The inpatient assessment should be within 48 hours if the patient is stable.
- Use the following non-invasive stress tests (see Chapter 16 for further details of each):
  - Exercise ECG.
  - Stress radionuclide myocardial perfusion imaging or stress cardiac magnetic resonance imaging.
  - Stress echocardiography.
  - Stress radionuclide ventriculography.
  - Positive features on the tests are suggestive of patients likely to suffer further re-infarction and adverse outcomes.

---

**MICRO-print**
**Chest pain + raised JVP/ankle oedema + systemic hypoperfusion + clear chest**
A *RV STEMI* due to RCA obstruction presents with ST segment elevation in V4R–V6R (on a right-sided chest leads ECG) and signs of acute RV failure and low output without pulmonary oedema. Management is by optimizing preload with fluids and minimizing afterload using nitroprusside or hydralazine, with a view to reperfusion.

---

**Summary of management of ACS (with ECG results known)**

| | STEMI | COMMON MANAGEMENT | UA/NSTEMI |
|---|---|---|---|
| Early medical | Clopidogrel 300 mg<br>Early ACEi post-reperfusion in 24 hours | $O_2$ if hypoxic<br>Aspirin 300 mg bolus<br>GTN infusion<br>Opiate pain relief<br>Beta-blockers<br>**High-dose statins** | Clopidogrel 300 mg for all but lowest risk<br>Calcium antagonists<br>**Anti-coagulants**<br>**GPI** |
| Early risk stratify | | | Use, e.g. TIMI score, GRACE score |
| Intervention | PCI<br>Thrombolysis<br>CABG | | Early conservative<br>Early coronary angiography ± PCI<br>CABG |
| Late risk stratify | Post-thrombolysis:<br>Inpatient or outpatient angiography<br>Electrophysiology studies | Exercise ECG<br>Stress perfusion imaging<br>Stress radionuclide ventriculography<br>Stress echocardiogram | Inpatient coronary angiography for those deemed at high risk with stress testing after early conservative management or with evidence of continuing ischaemia |

Cardiology and the cardiovascular system

| INTERVENTION | PERCUTANEOUS CORONARY INTERVENTION (PCI) | THROMBOLYSIS | CORONARY ARTERY BYPASS GRAFT (CABG) |
|---|---|---|---|
| Purpose | Treatment of a stenosis in the coronary circulation by: Flattening of an obstructing plaque Dilatation of the coronary artery Maintenance of lumen patency with a stent | To reperfuse the coronary arteries by clot dissolution in STEMI patients | Bypassing a stenosis using a graft to revascularize ischaemic myocardium Main benefit is symptom control Little prognostic benefit except in certain cases |
| Indications | STEMI NSTEMI/UA Stable angina | Chest pain with either one of the below: • New LBBB • ST segment elevation of 2 mm in 2 adjacent chest leads or 1 mm in 2 adjacent limb leads Within 60 minutes of an emergency call (call-to-needle time) Within 20 minutes of reaching hospital (door-to-needle time) | Persistent symptoms despite medical therapy in stable angina, additionally prognostic benefit if: • Left main stem disease with stenosis >50% even if asymptomatic • Triple vessel disease (LAD, left circumflex, right posterior descending) • Two-vessel disease including the LAD After ACS only if persistent symptoms despite medical therapy and in those with mechanical complications requiring surgery |

*Continued*

| INTERVENTION | PERCUTANEOUS CORONARY INTERVENTION (PCI) | THROMBOLYSIS | CORONARY ARTERY BYPASS GRAFT (CABG) |
|---|---|---|---|
| Contraindications | MI with complications requiring surgery<br>LMS coronary artery disease requiring CABG<br>Inability to administer anti-coagulants due to active major bleeding<br>Lack of vascular access | Various guidelines exist including those from the European Society of Cardiology, 2008<br>Examples of absolute contraindications include previous haemorrhagic stroke, major trauma or surgery in the past 3 weeks and central nervous system trauma or neoplasm | This is a major surgery and the risk of mortality and morbidity may be too great in a cohort of patients |
| Complications | Acute MI (risk 1:100): vessel spasm, occlusion, thrombus, dissection ± need for CABG<br>Ventricular tachyarrhythmias<br>Coronary artery perforation<br>Stroke (risk 1:1000)<br>Infection, haematoma, pseudoaneurysm, dissection at site of vascular access<br>Anaphylactic reaction to contrast agent | Haemorrhagic stroke (0.5–1.0% risk)<br>Bleeding at site of injection or elsewhere<br>Hypotension or anaphylaxis (seen mainly with streptokinase)<br>Reperfusion arrhythmias | Death<br>Vascular: MI, stroke (embolic or ischaemic due to hypotension) or systemic emboli<br>Infective mediastinitis (staphylococci, anaerobes)<br>Renal failure or respiratory failure<br>Ventricular tachyarrhythmias and atrial fibrillation postoperatively<br>Cognitive short-term decline (memory disturbance) |

*Continued*

Cardiology and the cardiovascular system

| INTERVENTION | PERCUTANEOUS CORONARY INTERVENTION (PCI) | THROMBOLYSIS | CORONARY ARTERY BYPASS GRAFT (CABG) |
|---|---|---|---|
| Further management | Dual therapy with aspirin (75 mg) and clopidogrel (75 mg) or other, e.g. ticagrelor is necessary for 1 month with a bare metal stent and usually for 12 months with a drug-eluting stent due to risk of late stent thrombosis<br><br>Aspirin will be continued lifelong as part of secondary prevention in CAD<br><br>Early discharge possible | Patients with recurrent chest pain symptoms after completed STEMI should be considered for elective intervention by angiography followed by either angioplasty or CABG<br><br>Efficacy may be evaluated by symptom relief, ST segment elevation resolution<br><br>Lack of resolution may need a rescue PCI | |

# 3.5 COMPLICATIONS OF MYOCARDIAL INFARCTION (SEE FIGURE 3.6)

| EARLY COMPLICATIONS | AETIOLOGY |
|---|---|
| **Conductive: arrhythmias** | |
| • Early VT and VF in the first 48 hours<br>• Incidence most common within hours of infarct<br>• Bradyarrhythmias may need pacing<br>• Risk is independent of infarct size<br>• Ventricular ectopics are common and benign | • Ischaemic myocyte metabolism disturbance<br>• Re-entry circuits form at the junction of necrotic and viable myocardium<br>• Increased sympathetic activation<br>• Changes in serum electrolytes |
| **Circulatory: cardiogenic shock** | |
| • Systolic BP <90 mmHg refractory to fluid therapy<br>• Treat with inotropes and temporary intra-aortic balloon pump | • Large LV or RV infarct results in acute HF<br>• Mechanical rupture of myocardium/acute valve incompetence |
| **Inflammatory: pericarditis** | |
| • Common >12 hours post-MI<br>• Treat with high-dose aspirin | • Inflammatory reaction to necrotic myocardium most common post-STEMI |
| **Mechanical: myocardial rupture** | |
| • Usually presents 3–5 days post-MI<br>• Assess for new murmurs and use echocardiograms<br>  • Papillary muscle rupture<br>  • Ventricular septal rupture<br>  • LV free wall rupture<br>• May require surgical repair and CABG<br>• Can cause acute cardiogenic shock or cardiac tamponade if free wall rupture | • Necrosis of myocytes can lead to myocardial thinning and eventual rupture<br>• Septal rupture more common in anterolateral infarcts and usually due to a STEMI<br>• Papillary muscle rupture can cause acute mitral regurgitation and acute heart failure |
| **Embolic: mural thrombus and embolism** | |
| • May be detected with echocardiograms<br>• Importance of anti-coagulation post-MI | • Thrombus formation due to blood stasis from wall dyskinesis or arrhythmias |

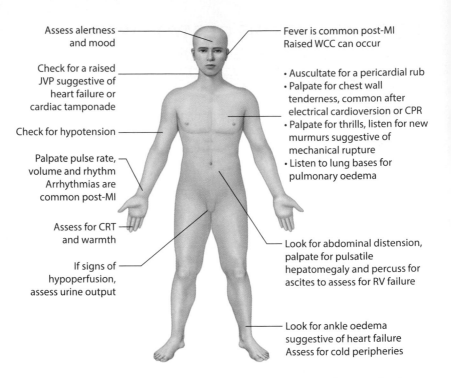

Assess alertness and mood

Check for a raised JVP suggestive of heart failure or cardiac tamponade

Check for hypotension

Palpate pulse rate, volume and rhythm Arrhythmias are common post-MI

Assess for CRT and warmth

If signs of hypoperfusion, assess urine output

Fever is common post-MI Raised WCC can occur

- Auscultate for a pericardial rub
- Palpate for chest wall tenderness, common after electrical cardioversion or CPR
- Palpate for thrills, listen for new murmurs suggestive of mechanical rupture
- Listen to lung bases for pulmonary oedema

Look for abdominal distension, palpate for pulsatile hepatomegaly and percuss for ascites to assess for RV failure

Look for ankle oedema suggestive of heart failure Assess for cold peripheries

**Figure 3.6** Clinical examination of the post-MI patient to assess for complications.

## MICRO-facts

The 6-month mortality from the time of hospital admission is 12% for a STEMI, 10% for NSTEMI and 5% for UA (data from GRACE multinational study, BMJ 2006).

Arrhythmic complications are the most common cause of early post-MI death.

**MICRO-reference**

Fox et al. Prediction of risk of death and myocardial infarction in the six months after presentation with acute coronary syndrome: prospective multinational observational study (GRACE). *BMJ*. 2006; 333: 1091–1094.

| LATE COMPLICATIONS | AETIOLOGY |
|---|---|
| **Conductive: late arrhythmias** | |
| • AF is common post-MI<br>• Ventricular ectopics or VT<br>• Adverse prognostic indicator associated with heart failure | • Formation of fibrotic tissue alters conduction and results in re-entry circuits |
| **Mechanical: chronic heart failure** | |
| • Adverse prognostic factor | • Large infarction causes pump dyskinesis |
| **Mechanical: ventricular aneurysm** | |
| • Less common with reperfusion therapy<br>• ST segment elevation persisting over 6 weeks is suggestive of aneurysmal formation<br>• Can be complicated by thrombus formation | • Due to myocardial necrosis leading to wall thinning and scar tissue formation |
| **Inflammatory: Dressler's syndrome** | |
| • Rare in context of current practice (early reperfusion therapy)<br>• Appears at 2–3 weeks post-MI (compare with post-MI pericarditis)<br>• Treat with high-dose aspirin | • Autoimmune aetiology caused by antibody formation to new myocardial antigens |

## MICRO-facts

A **true ventricular aneurysm** is due to dilatation of the ventricular wall containing all three heart layers and scar tissue. It occurs due to myocardial damage as a consequence of ischaemia post-MI. A **false ventricular aneurysm (pseudoaneurysm)** is walled by the pericardium and occurs due to ventricular free wall rupture contained by the surrounding pericardium.

# 3.6 LONG-TERM MANAGEMENT

Peri-discharge checklist and secondary prevention

## RISK STRATIFICATION

- Stress testing for patients who have not undergone invasive management with angiography (better delayed for 4–6 weeks post-infarction)
- Echocardiogram to assess residual LV function and to help direct drug management

Cardiology and the cardiovascular system

## LIFESTYLE MODIFICATION DISCUSSION

| Dietary changes | |
|---|---|
| Recommendation | Five portions of fruit and vegetable daily, two portions of oily fish weekly (omega-3 fatty acids), low sodium diet, less saturated fat |
| Benefits | Reduction in weight reduces CAD risk |
| | Insufficient evidence supporting reduction in mortality |
| **Alcohol limitation** | |
| Recommendation | Maximum 21 units weekly for males, 14 units weekly for females |
| Benefits | Reduction in malnutrition and alcohol-associated pathology |
| **Physical activity** | |
| Recommendation | Long-term aim for 30–60 minutes daily or until symptoms (e.g. dyspnoea) |
| Benefits | Exercise helps cardiac rehabilitation; regular exercise induces vagal tone which reduces basal heart rate and is beneficial |
| **Smoking cessation** | |
| Recommendation | Appropriate referral to quit smoking services |
| Benefits | Smoking cessation post-MI reduces mortality by approximately 33% |
| | An immediate decrease in incidence of ACS is observable with cessation |

## MEDICATION REVIEW

All the medications below reduce recurrence of cardiac events and mortality:

| **Anti-platelet** | Low-dose aspirin to be continued indefinitely in the absence of contraindications |
|---|---|
| | Dual therapy with clopidogrel or similar may be added for up to 12 months |
| **Beta-blocker** | Especially if there is any LV impairment post-MI |
| **Statin, ACEi** | Especially beneficial in patients with diabetes |
| | Evidence suggests risk reduction is independent of blood pressure lowering effect |
| | Especially beneficial in patients with diabetes and those with LV impairment |
| **Aldosterone antagonists** | Evidence suggests that risk is reduced in those patients who have had a cardiac event with LV dysfunction and congestive heart failure or diabetes mellitus |

Cardiology and the cardiovascular system

- **Influenza vaccination** is recommended but there is insufficient evidence supporting its role in hospital admission reduction due to heart disease.
- **Adequate diabetic control**, intensive HbA1c control does not necessarily decrease mortality.
- **BP control** aims <140/90 mmHg, and <130/80 mmHg in diabetes or chronic kidney disease.

---

**MICRO-print**

Evidence from the PLATO trial reviewed by NICE suggests that **ticagrelor** (see Section 17.5) in combination with aspirin for 12 months post-ACS may be more effective than clopidogrel + aspirin at preventing recurrence of vascular events.

---

## CARDIAC REHABILITATION

- A programme undertaken under the supervision of medical and allied healthcare staff that includes supervised exercise training and building the confidence of the patient post-ACS.

## PATIENT EDUCATION

*Physical exertion*
- Increase slowly, take recommendations from the cardiac rehabilitation team.

*Returning to the workplace*
- Return to work at 4–6 weeks post-MI if sedentary job.
- Return to work at 3 months post-MI if heavy manual job.

*Driving*
- Post-uncomplicated PCI, patients may resume driving after 1 week provided LVF >40%.
- Post-CABG, patients may resume driving after 1 month.
- Post-ACS without reperfusion therapy, driving may be resumed after 1 month.
- Driving must be discontinued if anginal symptoms appear at rest.

*Mental health*
- 1/3 of patients have evidence of depression post-MI.
- Up to 20% of hospitalized patients with MI have evidence supporting major depression.

*Sexual health*
- Sexual intercourse can be resumed 4 weeks post-MI.

*Travel insurer*
- Advice has been issued by the British Cardiovascular Society.

Cardiology and the cardiovascular system

- Advise the patient to contact airline and travel insurance if in doubt:
  - Post-ACS: low-risk patients can fly after 3 days, high-risk patients should defer travel until condition is stable.
  - Post-elective PCI: patients can fly after 2 days.
  - Post-elective CABG: if uncomplicated, patients can fly after 10 days.

---

**MICRO-references**

The DVLA has specific guidance regarding presentations of coronary artery disease and driving (https://www.gov.uk/health-conditions-and-driving). The civil aviation authority has also issued guidance on cardiovascular disease and air travel (https://www.caa.co.uk/default.aspx/default.aspx?catid=2497&pagetype=90).

---

**MICRO-case**

A 60-year-old man presented to the ED with sudden-onset central chest pain radiating to the jaw after climbing a flight of stairs. In the ambulance, he received oxygen and aspirin. The pain persisted despite sublingual GTN and IV diamorphine. The ECG showed 3 mm ST depression and T wave inversion in V1, V2 and V3 with additional T wave inversion in all other leads. Given the presence of ST depression in the antero-septal leads, an additional ECG with posterior leads V7, V8 and V9 was recorded. It showed 2 mm ST segment elevation in these leads. A diagnosis of posterior STEMI with haemodynamic stability was made and explained to the patient. Within the hour he was transferred to a regional centre for primary PCI. The blocked circumflex artery was stented with a bare-metal stent and a repeat ECG showed resolution of the ST segment elevation and the development of Q waves. He was commenced on dual anti-platelet therapy, bisoprolol, atorvastatin and an ACE inhibitor. The patient was monitored on telemetry that initially showed short runs of non-sustained VT, with no further arrhythmias in the subsequent days. He remained chest pain-free and was reviewed daily for complications such as heart failure. An echocardiogram was performed which showed regional wall motion abnormalities with mild overall left ventricular systolic dysfunction. He was advised to stop smoking, given information on services which could support him with this, and enrolled in a cardiac rehabilitation programme.

**Points to consider:**

- Note that ST elevation MI requires urgent diagnosis for early reperfusion.
- It is possible to miss a posterior or right-sided STEMI as traditional chest leads do not pick these up. The presence of ST depression in leads V1–V3 suggests a posterior STEMI.
- Complications in the post-MI patient include arrhythmias and heart failure.

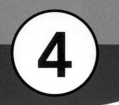

# 4      Acute heart failure

## 4.1 AETIOLOGY

### CARDIAC CAUSES (SEE FIGURE 4.1)

- Acute MI and any subsequent septal rupture
- Valvular dysfunction:
    - Chronic and progressive left-sided valve stenosis or regurgitation (e.g. rheumatic valve disease) – acute decompensation of a chronic disorder
    - Acute valve rupture and regurgitation
    - Chordae tendinae rupture
    - Papillary muscle rupture

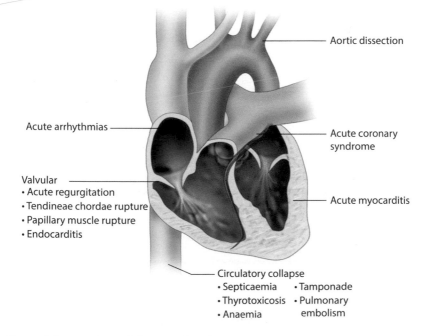

Figure 4.1  Acute heart failure aetiology by anatomy.

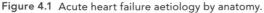

- Infective endocarditis
- Aortic dissection leading to aortic regurgitation
- Acute myocarditis
- Acute arrhythmias

## RESTRICTION OF VENTRICULAR FILLING

- Constrictive pericarditis
- Cardiac tamponade

## INCREASED PRELOAD OR AFTERLOAD

- Uncontrolled hypertension
- Worsening valvular stenosis
- PE (right-sided heart failure)
- Systemic volume overload, e.g. renal failure

## SYSTEMIC FACTORS ACUTELY INCREASING DEMAND ON PUMP

- Septicaemia
- Anaemia
- Thyrotoxicosis
- Post-surgery or trauma

## DRUGS

- Causing side effects of cardiac arrhythmias, heart block, hypertension, fluid retention and direct cardiac muscle toxicity

## TOXINS

- Alcohol
- Heavy metals
- Acute cytokine release as in multi-system trauma or septicaemia

# 4.2 SYMPTOMS AND SIGNS

> **MICRO-facts**
>
> Acute decompensated chronic heart failure may present with symptoms of worsening NYHA score.

- Signs of pre-existing heart failure may be present
- Look for symptoms of precipitants such as:
  - Chest pain (indicating acute MI, PE or aortic dissection)
  - Palpitations (arrhythmias)

- Look for signs of precipitants such as:
  - Fever in sepsis
  - New murmurs in valvular regurgitation

|  | SYMPTOMS | SIGNS |
|---|---|---|
| Pulmonary congestion | Dyspnoea<br>Wheeze<br>Orthopnoea<br>Paroxysmal nocturnal dyspnoea<br>Agitation, sweating | Peripheral and central cyanosis<br>Use of accessory muscles of breathing<br>Tachypnoea<br>Fine inspiratory crepitations<br>Pink frothy sputum |
| Systemic congestion | Swollen ankles | Raised JVP<br>Hepatomegaly and ascites<br>Peripheral oedema |
| Reduced systemic perfusion | Altered mental status | Tachycardia<br>Hypotension<br>Cold, moist, cyanosed peripheries<br>Poor capillary refill<br>Oliguria |
| Chronic heart failure | Fatigue | Pulsus alternans<br>Displaced apex beat due to cardiomegaly<br>Ventricular heave<br>Added heart sound – S3 (gallop rhythm)<br>Cachexia |

| Pulmonary congestion THINK Pulmonary oedema? | **Definition?** Fluid accumulation within alveoli and lung interstitium<br>**Why can it occur in acute heart failure (AHF)** Due to increased capillary hydrostatic pressure resulting in a transudate in the lungs |
|---|---|
| Poor perfusion THINK Cardiogenic shock? | **Definition?** Persistent (>30 minutes) hypotension with SBP <90 mmHg with a reduced cardiac index and an elevated LV filling pressure (pulmonary capillary wedge pressure [PCWP] >18 mmHg)<br>**Why can it occur in AHF?** Due to ineffective cardiac output |

---

**MICRO-print**
**Causes of non-cardiogenic pulmonary oedema?**
Increased capillary permeability, as in acute respiratory distress syndrome (ARDS)
Decreased intravascular oncotic pressure as in hypoalbuminaemia of hepatic failure or nephrotic syndrome

Cardiology and the cardiovascular system

## 4.3 INVESTIGATIONS

### AIM TO

- Diagnose AHF
- Rule out non-cardiogenic causes for pulmonary oedema
- Identify precipitants

| Laboratory tests | FBC | Precipitating factors such as anaemia or infection |
|---|---|---|
| | U&E | May show renal impairment<br>Use baseline electrolytes to monitor therapy side effects<br>Dilutional hyponatraemia may be present |
| | BNP | BNP secreted by ventricles in response to stretch |
| | CK, CK-MB, troponins | To assess precipitation by ACS<br>Troponins may be mildly elevated in AHF without acute MI |
| | CRP | Normal CRP may be useful in ruling out infection, acute lung injury and ARDS |
| **ABG** | $\downarrow P_aO_2$, $\downarrow P_aCO_2$ if severe oedema<br>$\uparrow P_aCO_2$ if hypoventilation and respiratory acidosis may be present | |
| **ECG** | Sinus tachycardia<br>Look for pre-existing or precipitating abnormalities such as LV hypertrophy, arrhythmias, bundle branch block or ischaemia | |
| **Imaging** | CXR | Look for signs of pulmonary oedema (see Figure 4.2)<br>Exclude pneumothorax and lobar pneumonia |
| | Echo | Look for LV dysfunction, dilatation and pericardial effusion<br>Search for precipitant: valve regurgitation, septal defect |
| **Other** | Clotting, INR, glucose, TFT, septic screen | Consider if appropriate |
| **Severe AHF** | Swan-Ganz catheter | PCWP elevation >20 mmHg suggests acute pulmonary oedema and may help to differentiate between cardiac and non-cardiac causes of pulmonary oedema |

Cardiology and the cardiovascular system

## MICRO-facts

An urgent echocardiogram is the single most useful test to determine the diagnosis and cause of AHF.

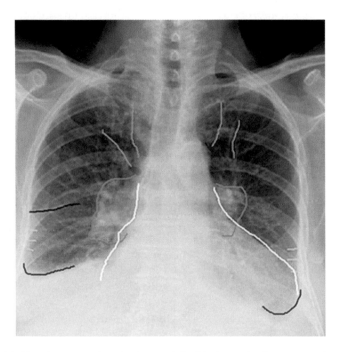

**Figure 4.2** The above is a chest radiograph highlighting the features evident in acute heart failure as outlined below.

### AKCUTE pulmonary oedema

**A**lveolar oedema

**K**erley B lines

**C**ardiomegaly

**U**pper lobe diversion

**T**ransudate in fissures

**E**ffusion (pleural)

# 4.4 MANAGEMENT OF ACUTE HEART FAILURE

## MONITOR AND MANAGE

- **ABC and resuscitation:** acute pulmonary oedema is a medical emergency.
- **Call for help if appropriate:** senior help, anaesthetist on-call, consider informing CCU/ ITU.
- **Sit patient upright if possible.**
- **15 L oxygen via a non-rebreathable mask**, caution in patients with COPD.
- **Continuous cardiac monitoring** and cardioversion for unstable arrhythmia.
- **Secure venous access** and send bloods for investigation.
- **Initiate pharmacological treatment.**

| Diamorphine | 2.5 mg IV | ↓ Anxiety, ↓ dyspnoea and ↓ preload by venodilation |
|---|---|---|
| Metoclopramide | 10 mg IV | Anti-emetic for opiate-induced nausea |
| Furosemide or bumetanide | 40–120 mg IV<br>1 mg IV | Primarily ↓ afterload by venodilation within 30 minutes<br>↓ Preload by diuresis<br>↓ Renal flow by ↑ renal prostaglandin synthesis<br>Intestinal oedema ↓ absorption of oral furosemide<br>Bumetanide is better absorbed through an oedematous intestine |
| Thiazide or thiazide-like diuretic | | In resistant peripheral oedema: loop + thiazide diuretic<br>Thiazide diuretic if creatinine clearance is >30 mL/min, metolazone is unaffected by creatinine clearance |

- **Urinary catheter insertion** allows accurate monitoring of output for fluid balance.
- Consider the use of **continuous positive airway pressure** (CPAP) if necessary:
    - It improves alveolar ventilation and re-expands flooded alveoli.
    - It decreases heart rate due to parasympathetic stimulation in inflated lungs.

- It decreases preload and afterload by decreasing the cardiac transmural pressure (pressure difference between the inside of the heart and the intrathoracic pressure), thereby easing the work of the heart and myocardial $O_2$ demand.

## INITIATE IMMEDIATE INVESTIGATIONS

- ABG
- Plain chest radiograph (CXR)
- ECG
- Obtain an echocardiogram as soon as possible

---

### MICRO-facts

The CXR may lack signs of congestion in over 15% of patients with AHF.

---

## ASSESS

- Respiratory distress
- Haemodynamic status
- Precipitating causes

### Poor prognostic factors

- Low systolic BP
- Ischaemic heart disease
- Raised cardiac troponin
- Increased serum creatinine and urea
- Elevated BNP
- Hyponatraemia
- Co-morbidities

---

**MICRO-print**
Many different clinical prediction models using these prognostic factors have been studied to stratify AHF patients into risk categories. An example is the risk stratification tool based on the US Acute Decompensated Heart Failure National Registry (ADHERE).

---

Cardiology and the cardiovascular system

Additional management of AHF

| | |
|---|---|
| **RESPIRATORY** | Aim SpO$_2$ >95% (if no history of type II respiratory failure)<br>• If signs of respiratory distress persist, consider non-invasive ventilation in the form of CPAP. This therapy:<br>  • Improves alveolar ventilation and reduces myocardial O$_2$ consumption:<br>  • Does not improve short-term or long-term survival<br>  • Indicated in cooperative patients with<br>    – Continued dyspnoea<br>    – Persistent hypoxaemia<br>    – Persistent acidosis<br>    – No hypotension |
| **HAEMODYNAMICS** | **Hypotensive** (systolic BP <90 mmHg) constitutes <5% of cases of AHF.<br>• Cardiogenic shock is the most common cause.<br>• Cardiogenic shock management and mechanical assist devices such as intra-aortic balloon counter pulsation (IABP) (see p. 57).<br><br>**Normotensive** or **hypertensive** (systolic BP >140 mmHg)<br>• Add nitrates to ↓preload, ↓afterload and ↑coronary perfusion by vasodilatation.<br>• Beware of hypotension as a side effect:<br>  • Sublingual GTN spray (2 puffs) or IV GTN infusion (1–10 mg/hour)<br>  • IV sodium nitroprusside is only used in severe hypertensive AHF<br>    – Consider an arterial line for monitoring BP<br>  • Isosorbide dinitrate (1 mg/h)<br>  • IV nesiritide, a BNP analogue, has not been shown to significantly improve mortality and dyspnoea (not licensed in the UK)<br>• If BP <100 mmHg and peripheries are cool, consider the use of inotropic therapy. |
| **TREAT CAUSE** | • **Reperfusion** interventions for acute MI<br>• **Emergency surgery** indicated for papillary muscle, chordae tendinae, septal defect and free wall rupture and dissecting abdominal aneurysm<br>• **Pericardiocentesis** for cardiac tamponade<br>• **Medical treatment** for septicaemia, anaemia, thyrotoxicosis, endocarditis and other precipitating causes |

Continue to monitor symptoms and signs, BP, work of breathing, O$_2$ saturation, cardiac activity, fluid balance, daily weights

## 4.5 CARDIOGENIC SHOCK

**ABC, diagnose, monitor and manage**

### DIAGNOSIS

• Inadequate end-organ perfusion due to cardiac dysfunction
• Diagnosed at the bedside clinically and confirmed physiologically

Physiological criteria

• Low cardiac index (<1.8 L/mm/m$^2$)
• Elevated LV filling pressure (PCWP >18 mmHg)

> **MICRO-facts**
>
> The cardiac index is the cardiac output per unit of body surface.

Clinical criteria

- Hypotension (SBP <90 mmHg) is persistent (>30 minutes)
- Signs of tissue hypoperfusion:
  - Cold, moist peripheries
  - Low urinary output
  - Altered mentation

## MONITOR AND ASSESS

- Haemodynamics:
  - **Arterial line** for arterial BP and serial ABG
  - **Central venous line** for venous oxygen saturation ($SVO_2$) and venous access
  - **Swan-Ganz catheter** to be considered
  - **Urinary catheter** to measure urine output
- LV dysfunction: order an urgent echocardiogram
- Angiography: to consider revascularization – remember that acute MI is the most common cause of cardiogenic shock

---

**MICRO-print**
**Aims in cardiogenic shock:**

- Warm peripheries
- Systolic BP >90 mmHg
- PCWP 16–18 mmHg

Prognosis is poor

---

### MANAGEMENT

- Identify and reverse acute arrhythmias and electrolyte imbalances.
- Use:
  - *Pharmacological* therapy to increase cardiac output
  - *Mechanical* support systems (IABP and ventricular assist devices)
- As a bridge to:
  - *Reperfusion* interventions (PCI and CABG)
  - *Surgical* repair of ruptured free wall or papillary muscle
  - *Heart transplant* (rarely)

Pharmacological therapy

- Relies on inotropic drug infusions to increase cardiac contractility via $\beta_1$ receptors.
- These drugs often have vasopressor effects mediated by $\alpha$ adrenergic receptors.

Cardiology and the cardiovascular system

| Dobutamine | Dopamine | Epinephrine |
|---|---|---|
| When SBP >80 mmHg | When SBP <80 mmHg | Alternative to high-dose dopamine |

Provides renal vasodilatation

→

Inotropes with increasing vasopressor effect so consider adding a vasodilator

### Intra-aortic balloon counterpulsation (IABP)

- IABP is a *temporary* mechanical device providing circulatory support and improving myocardial ischaemia.
- IABP insertion should ideally be done in a catheter laboratory to ensure sterility and to allow the use of fluoroscopy.

*Working principles (see Figure 4.3):*

- A 34–40 cm deflated balloon is inserted at the femoral artery site.
- Once inflated, it sits in the proximal descending aorta just below the arch.
- Timed using surface ECGs, the balloon is inflated immediately after aortic valve closure marking the start of diastole and deflated at the end of diastole.

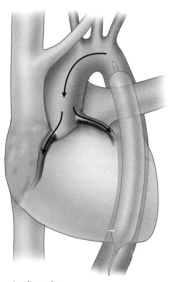

In diastole
Balloon inflation pushes blood into coronary arteries

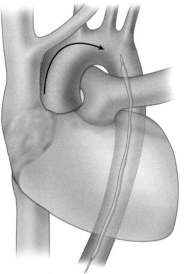

In systole
Balloon deflation reduces afterload and encourages systemic flow

**Figure 4.3** IABP working mechanism.

| Effect of inflation start of diastole | Distally blood is displaced towards the systemic circulation | Increased cardiac output |
|---|---|---|
| | Proximally blood is encouraged to flow through the coronary circulation (diastolic augmentation) | Increased myocardial perfusion |
| Effect of deflation end of diastole | Reduces afterload | Increased cardiac index Decreased myocardial O$_2$ use |

## INDICATIONS

- Cardiogenic shock
- Severe pulmonary oedema
- Intractable angina
- To bridge patients for:
  - Reperfusion intervention post-MI
  - Surgical correction for acute mitral regurgitation or septal rupture post-MI
  - Cardiac transplant

| ABSOLUTE CONTRAINDICATIONS | RELATIVE CONTRAINDICATIONS |
|---|---|
| • Significant aortic regurgitation<br>• Aortic dissection<br>• Lack of anticipation of recovery | • Abdominal aortic aneurysm<br>• Tachyarrhythmias<br>• Severe peripheral vascular disease |

## MICRO-facts

**Remember:** Patients with an IABP are immobile and may be at risk of thromboembolism, making anti-coagulation a necessary consideration.

### MICRO-print

*Considerations during insertion*

- Patients need anti-coagulation with heparin
- IABP is less effective in tachycardic patients

*Considerations during removal*

- Prepare atropine
- Patients may require weaning off IABP

*Complications*

- Leg ischaemia
- Arterial embolism

Cardiology and the cardiovascular system

# 5 Chronic heart failure

- Usually a progressive disorder, but there are some rare causes of reversible heart failure.
- Due to a damaged heart that weakens gradually and is eventually unable to supply the metabolic demands of the tissues.
- Management is focused on reducing symptoms, optimizing contractile cardiac function and slowing progression.
- Five-year survival is around 50% and treatment delays death.

## 5.1 CLASSIFICATION

### ACUTE VERSUS CHRONIC

- Symptoms depend on the speed of onset.
- Acute heart failure causes acute-onset dyspnoea and pulmonary oedema from LV failure (this stage is before physiological compensation has occurred).
- In chronic heart failure (CHF), there is objective evidence of contractile dysfunction but symptoms are controlled by drug therapy.

### RIGHT VERSUS LEFT

- RV failure is characterized by reduced pulmonary arterial flow resulting in venous engorgement elevating central venous pressure, hepatic congestion and peripheral oedema.
- LV failure results from the inability to pump sufficient blood into the systemic circulation.
- LV failure leads to high LV residual volume and pressure, causing reduced trans-mitral inflow and increasing back pressure in the pulmonary venous circulation, eventually resulting in extrusion of fluid in the alveoli, causing pulmonary oedema.

### SYSTOLIC VERSUS DIASTOLIC

- About 50% of patients suffering from heart failure have impaired LV systolic function.

- The other half has symptoms of heart failure but preserved systolic function – diastolic heart failure.
- Diastolic dysfunction occurs especially in obese, hypertensive and diabetic patients.

## HIGH OUTPUT VERSUS LOW OUTPUT

- High output heart failure occurs when there is persistently high venous return, e.g. arterio-venous fistula.
- Low output heart failure is much more common and results in lower than normal cardiac output and blood pressure, with a subsequent compensatory tachycardia.

# 5.2 PATHOPHYSIOLOGY AND PRESENTATION OF CHF

## CAUSES OF CHF

LV failure can be caused by three different mechanisms:

- **Preload** – increased LV volume causes LV dilatation with associated hypertrophy:
  - Blood or IV fluid overload (iatrogenic)
  - Mitral valve regurgitation
  - Aortic valve regurgitation
- **Afterload** – increased systemic pressure that increases cardiac work resulting in LV hypertrophy:
  - Hypertension
  - Aortic stenosis
  - Pulmonary hypertension from respiratory diseases that results in RV failure
- **Direct damage of the ventricles:**
  - Ischaemic heart disease and myocardial infarction – causes 60% of all cases of CHF
  - Cardiomyopathies
  - Drug and alcohol toxicity
  - Pericardial disease, which also affects the myocardium
  - Congenital heart disease

## PATHOPHYSIOLOGY OF HEART FAILURE

- Failure of the LV eventually leads to increased pressures in the pulmonary artery, RV and RA producing symptoms of both pulmonary and systemic venous congestion, otherwise known as **congestive cardiac failure**.
- Compensatory neuro-hormonal effects are triggered when heart failure occurs, usually prompted by a fall in cardiac output.

- Initially supportive (designed to increase blood volume and pressure), but eventually are maladaptive and lead to worsening heart failure.
- Decompensation occurs when these changes cannot maintain cardiac output and BP.

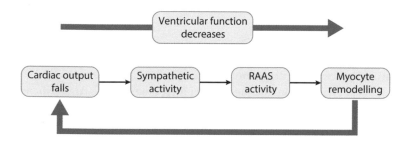

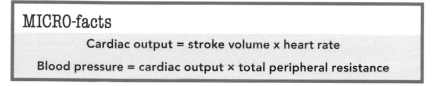

---

## MICRO-facts

**Cardiac output = stroke volume x heart rate**

**Blood pressure = cardiac output × total peripheral resistance**

---

### Starling's Law

- Starling's Law describes the relationship between preload (or myocardial stretch) and stroke volume (contraction power) (see Figure 5.1):
  - The power of myocardial contraction increases proportionally to the volume of end-diastolic blood in the ventricle.
  - Beyond a particular point increased volume will lead to reduced contraction.

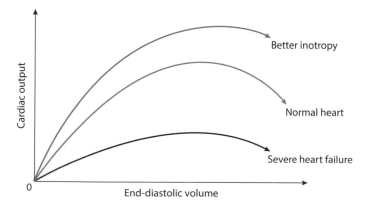

**Figure 5.1** Starling's curve.

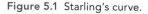

Cardiology and the cardiovascular system

*How does it go wrong?*

- Chronic increase in preload is thought to stretch the myofibrils excessively:
  - They become unable to respond to further changes in pressure.
- Persistently elevated diastolic pressure in the LV is transmitted backwards sequentially to the atria, pulmonary vessels and right ventricles, causing congestive heart failure.

## Sympathetic system activation

- Increased pressure within the ventricles and a reduced cardiac output trigger baroreceptors and cardiopulmonary mechanoreceptors.
- Results in increased production of norepinephrine, which acts on adreno-receptors in the myocardium and vessel walls causing:
  - **Increased heart rate** (sinus tachycardia is a sign of heart failure) mediated by $\beta_1$ receptors
  - **Increased myocardial contraction strength** mediated by $\beta_1$ receptors
  - **Peripheral arterial vasoconstriction** (with preferential blood supply to the heart and brain at the expense of the skin, gastrointestinal system and kidneys) mediated by $\alpha$ receptors

*How does it go wrong?*

- Increased contraction strength and rate also increase myocardial energy demands.
- Increased peripheral resistance causes increased after load and therefore cardiac work.
  - This can exacerbate existing ischaemia and there is a risk of **ventricular tachycardia** or **sudden death**.

---

**MICRO-print**

**Beta-blockers** work on the beta adrenoreceptors and reduce the effects of sympathetic activation, thereby reducing contraction strength and rate (negatively inotropic and chronotropic, respectively). They have been proven to reduce morbidity and mortality and are now a first-line treatment in non-decompensated patients. However, beware as their effect on contraction rate and strength can initially worsen symptoms.

---

## RAAS (renin–angiotensin–aldosterone system) activation

- RAAS activation is the mechanism by which salt and water are retained to increase preload (see Figure 5.2).
- Triggered by:
  - Renal hypoperfusion
  - Reduced salt delivery to the distal tubule
  - Stimulation by the adrenergic system
- Cause renin to be released from the juxtaglomerular cells.

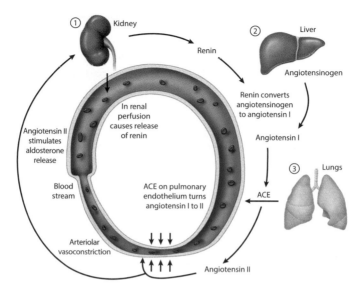

**Figure 5.2** RAAS activation.

### Angiotensin II
- Causes aldosterone release and has a direct effect on tubules to retain salt and water
- Potent vasoconstrictor
- Stimulates the thirst centres in the brain

### Aldosterone
- Increased sodium reabsorption

*How does it go wrong?*

- The retention of salt and water eventually causes fluid overload, with symptoms of peripheral oedema, hepatomegaly and weight gain.
- Chronic high levels of angiotensin II and aldosterone worsen LV systolic function by promoting hypertrophy and fibrosis within the vessels and myocardium.
- They increase norepinephrine levels and exacerbate activation of the sympathetic system.

---

**MICRO-print**

**Angiotensin-converting enzyme (ACE) inhibitors** and **angiotensin receptor blockers (ARBs)** block the RAAS and decrease production of angiotensin II and aldosterone. ACE inhibitors (ACEi) also increase bradykinin levels by stopping ACE-dependent bradykinin inactivation. Bradykinins have a vasodilating effect but are also responsible for a dry cough. ARBs do not block ACE production, so they can be used as an alternative for those who experience a dry cough with ACEi use.

---

Cardiology and the cardiovascular system

> ## MICRO-facts
> The negative effects of chronically elevated aldosterone levels continue even after treatment with ACEi's, as aldosterone production can continue independently of the RAAS. **Aldosterone antagonists** (spironolactone and eplerenone) cause a reduction in mortality in CHF, separate from their diuretic effect, and are therefore used as a second-line drug for moderate-to-severe CHF.

Ventricular remodelling

- Insults to the myocytes themselves and stress to the ventricular walls cause myocyte apoptosis, with secondary compensatory hypertrophy of living myocytes.
- The type of hypertrophy depends on the stresses on the ventricle wall:
  - Increased volume causes **wall dilatation** (reducing diastolic filling pressure).
  - Increased pressure leads to **wall thickening** (increases ventricular contraction strength).

*How does it go wrong?*

- Other elements of ventricular remodelling include collagen deposition in the extracellular matrix, which reduces ventricular compliance and causes myocyte loss.
- Scar replacement of dead myocytes leads to loss of cardiac relaxation and diastolic dysfunction.
- Hypertrophied myocytes have increased apoptosis and shorter life spans.
- The myocytes and therefore the ventricles fail to function as they should, demonstrating:
  - Poor contractility
  - Electrical and mechanical dyssynchrony

> **MICRO-print**
> **How does the body respond to these maladaptations?**
> There are several counter-regulatory mechanisms, most of which become blunted in CHF. Clinically, the most important is the production of **ANP** and **BNP (atrial and brain natriuretic peptides, respectively)** in response to stretching of the atria and ventricles. This increases excretion of salt and water and suppresses renin and aldosterone release. BNP production is particularly significant as it is used as a marker of severity in heart failure. If **serum natriuretic peptides** are at a normal level, then heart failure is unlikely to be the diagnosis.

SYMPTOMS AND SIGNS

- Result from maladaptive processes such as sympathetic overdrive or the reduced cardiac output of the failing heart, such as hypoperfusion of the kidneys, brain and skeletal muscles leading to oliguria, confusion, fatigue and weakness.

General examination

- Cachexia (reduced appetite and increased energy demands)
- Diaphoresis from sympathetic over-activity
- Sinus tachycardia
- Pulsus alterans – pulse that fluctuates between strong and weak from beat to beat (rare and only in end-stage heart failure)
- Hypotension

## MICRO-facts

**Revascularization**

There is no clear evidence that revascularization improves left ventricular systolic function or survival in CHF. As such, it should only be considered for treatment of symptoms of ischaemic heart disease (see Chapter 3), not for CHF of ischaemic aetiology without anginal symptoms.

- Peripheral cyanosis from poor peripheral circulation (sympathetic activation)
- Tachypnoea: in severe and end-stage heart failure a Cheyne–Stokes breathing pattern can appear, with a cyclical increase in depth and rate of breathing followed by a decrease in depth and rate, possibly with apnoeas (happens when circulation is slowed between the chemoreceptors responsible for breathing and the lungs)

## MICRO-facts

On examination look for signs of arrhythmia and valve disease as both can cause HF or result from HF. For example, mitral regurgitation can cause HF as a result of increased preload but can also occur if dilatation of the ventricle through ventricular remodelling has widened the annulus and stretched the papillary muscles.

Left heart failure

SYMPTOMS

- Dyspnoea
- Orthopnoea – dyspnoea when lying flat

- Paroxysmal nocturnal dyspnoea – sudden breathlessness disrupting sleep
- Nocturnal cough and wheeze
- Fatigue

## MICRO-facts

Dyspnoea occurs as hydrostatic forces from back pressure allow fluid to pass from the capillaries into the interstitium, reducing pulmonary compliance and compressing the walls of the small airways. On lying flat, the effect of gravity is reduced and venous return increases, increasing pulmonary congestion causing orthopnoea and nocturnal cough. The kidney also reabsorbs fluid at night, causing nocturia.

### Signs

- Peripheral cyanosis
- Tachycardia
- Relative hypotension
- S3 and S4 (rare) – gallop rhythm
- Inferiorly and laterally displaced apical beat and/or left ventricular heave depending on whether dilatation or enlargement is more prominent
- Wheeze (not universal)
- Bibasal crackles
- Dullness on percussion of lung bases due to pleural effusions

### MICRO-print

The NYHA classification of heart failure describes the level of functional impairment in patients with heart failure.

| NYHA CLASS | SYMPTOMS |
| --- | --- |
| I | No symptoms and no limitation in ordinary physical activity |
| II | Mild symptoms (e.g. shortness of breath or chest pain) and slight limitation during ordinary activity |
| III | Marked limitation in activity due to symptoms, even during less-than-ordinary activity, e.g. walking short distances (20–100 m)<br>Comfortable only at rest |
| IV | Experiences symptoms even while at rest<br>Mostly bed-bound patients |

## Right heart failure

- Most signs and symptoms are a result of systemic venous congestion.

### SYMPTOMS

- Foot, ankle and leg swelling
- Right upper quadrant pain as a result of an enlarged liver stretching the hepatic capsule
- Anorexia (from hepatic congestion)
- Abdominal swelling
- Weight gain

### SIGNS

- Elevated jugular venous pressure (JVP)
- Left parasternal heave representing RV dilatation and pressure overload
- Pitting oedema in the lower limbs or sacrum depending on position of patient
- Ascites
- Tender hepatomegaly

---

**MICRO-print**
**Kussmaul's sign** – the JVP rises on inspiration when it should normally fall. This is a sign of cardiac tamponade or restrictive cardiomyopathy (see p. 69).

---

# 5.3 INVESTIGATION OF CHF

- Diagnosis requires two major or one major and two minor criteria (Framingham study).
- Minor criteria are acceptable if they cannot be attributable to another disorder.

## FRAMINGHAM CRITERIA

| MAJOR CRITERIA | MINOR CRITERIA |
| --- | --- |
| Paroxysmal nocturnal dyspnoea | Bilateral ankle oedema |
| Neck vein distension | Nocturnal cough |
| Crackles | Dyspnoea on ordinary exertion |
| Radiographic cardiomegaly | Hepatomegaly |
| Acute pulmonary oedema | Pleural effusion |
| S3 gallop | Decrease in vital capacity by one third from maximum recorded |

*Continued*

Cardiology and the cardiovascular system

| MAJOR CRITERIA | MINOR CRITERIA |
|---|---|
| Increased central venous pressure (>16 cm H$_2$O at right atrium) | Tachycardia (heart rate >120 beats/min) |
| Hepatojugular reflex | |
| Weight loss >4.5 kg in 5 days in response to treatment | |

## DIAGNOSTIC TESTING

- The route of investigation depends on the past history of the patient:
  - If there is a previous MI, then echocardiogram is the diagnostic tool of choice.
  - If there is no history of MI, then first-line testing is with serum natriuretic peptides and an ECG.

### ECG

- No specific changes in heart failure.
- A completely normal ECG strongly predicts normal LV function and should encourage the search for other conditions causing the presenting symptoms.
- Otherwise look for AF, conduction defects, e.g. left bundle branch block (LBBB), and any evidence of previous MI.

### Natriuretic peptides

- Released by the ventricles in response to excessive stretch.
- Very high sensitivity but low specificity.
- With a normal ECG and normal natriuretic peptide levels, heart failure becomes an unlikely diagnosis.
- Raised natriuretic peptide levels should prompt a referral for echocardiography:
  - High levels are linked to a poor prognosis.

### Echocardiogram

- Echocardiogram can demonstrate cardiac dysfunction and valvular lesions.
- The degree of dysfunction can be defined as mild, moderate or severe.

## FURTHER TESTING

| Laboratory tests | FBC | Precipitating factors such as anaemia or infection |
|---|---|---|
| | U&E | May show renal impairment Use baseline electrolytes to monitor therapy side effects Dilutional hyponatraemia may be present |
| | LFT | Hepatic impairment due to congestion |
| | TFT | Hyper or hypothyroidism as a cause |
| | Viral titres Immunoglobulins | In individual cases where rare causes are suspected |
| **ECG** | Holter monitor Signal averaged ECG | At risk of ventricular arrhythmia +/– T wave alternans |
| **Imaging** | CXR | May show similar findings to acute heart failure |
| **Other** | Pulmonary function tests Angiography Nuclear scans Myocardial biopsy Cardiac MRI | To assess for co-morbid respiratory disease If an ischaemic cause is likely If an infiltrative aetiology is suspected |

# 5.4 MANAGEMENT OF CHF

## MICRO-facts

Clinical review of a patient with heart failure:

- Assess functional capacity, fluid status, cardiac rhythm (assessed by palpation of the pulse at minimum), cognitive and nutritional status.
- Review drug treatment – consider response to treatment and possible side effects.
- Measure urea, electrolytes, creatinine and estimated glomerular filtration rate.

Cardiology and the cardiovascular system

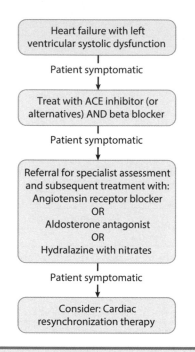

Patient should also receive:

- Treatment for comorbidities such as diabetes and hyperlipidaemia

- Lifestyle modification advice and education about the condition including access to rehabilitation, stop smoking and dietary advice

- Diuretic treatment in response to signs and symptoms of congestion and fluid retention

- An ICD (implantable cardiac defibrillator) can be considered when appropriate

**MICRO-reference**
National Institute for Health and Care Excellence. Chronic heart failure. NICE guidelines [CG108]. London: National Institute for Health and Care Excellence, 2010.

## FIRST-LINE TREATMENT

- **ACEi** both in symptomatic and asymptomatic heart failure:
  - Reduces symptoms
  - Reduces hospital admission
  - Prolongs life
- Consider **nitrates in combination with hydralazine** in patients with significant renal impairment (creatinine >20 μmol/L) who cannot use ACEi or ARBs.
- **Beta-blockers:**
  - Reduce symptoms
  - Prolong life
- Three drugs are licensed for use in heart failure:
  - **Bisoprolol** and **carvedilol** (for any grade of heart failure)
  - **Nebivolol** (for mild or moderate heart failure in patient >70 years old)

- Permanent pacing should be considered for patients whose beta-blocker therapy is limited by symptomatic bradycardia or AV block.

---

**MICRO-print**

Both beta-blockers and ACEi's can cause severe hypotension so a 'start low, go slow' approach is required. If hypotension is a problem:

- Check fluid levels – if volume depleted reduce diuretic therapy
- If euvolaemic consider stopping any vasodilating drugs
- Consider spreading the doses of drugs which cause hypotension
- Give the drug before bedtime

---

## FURTHER MANAGEMENT

- A third drug can be added for patients who remain symptomatic after two first-line drugs:
  - **Aldosterone antagonist** (for moderate-to-severe heart failure)
  - **Angiotensin receptor blocker** – specifically candesartan (for mild-to-moderate heart failure)
  - **Isosorbide nitrate with hydralazine** (moderate-to-severe, especially in patients of Afro-Caribbean origin)
- If the patient is still symptomatic after three drugs, **digoxin** may be used:
  - Improvement in exercise tolerance and symptoms
  - Reduction in the number of admission for acute exacerbations
  - No prolongation of life

---

**MICRO-print**
**Be careful of potassium**

- Loop and thiazide diuretics may cause hypokalaemia.
- Aldosterone antagonists, ACEi and ARBs can cause hyperkalaemia.
- Both hyperkalaemia and hypokalaemia can lead to arrhythmias and death.

---

## MICRO-facts

**Diuretics** can be used at any point in the course of HF for symptoms of fluid overload. Loop diuretics are the first choice. The options include **bumetanide, furosemide** and **torsemide**. In more severe cases, a thiazide (bendroflumethiazide) diuretic or metolazone (a thiazide-like diuretic) can be added. When this combination is added to the loop diuretic, there is an added risk of electrolyte abnormalities and dehydration.

## 5.5 DEVICES

- Half of patients die from sudden arrhythmic death (usually ventricular fibrillation/ventricular tachycardia although asystole may also occur).
- The remaining half die from low output heart failure and hence multi-organ failure.
- In some patients with heart failure, there is disordered intracardiac conduction, and therapy aimed at resynchronizing the ventricles may improve cardiac function.
- Resynchronization can occur with either:
  - CRT-P (CRT with pacemaker) or
  - CRT-D (CRT with implantable cardioverter defibrillator) devices (see Figure 5.3)

NICE recommends implantable cardioverter defibrillators (ICDs) for patients with symptoms classed III or below on the NYHA classification and who are at high risk of serious shockable ventricular arrhythmias, such as those who have:

  - Survived a VT or VF cardiac arrest
  - Sustained VT causing haemodynamic compromise or syncope
  - Sustained VT with no compromise but LVEF <35%

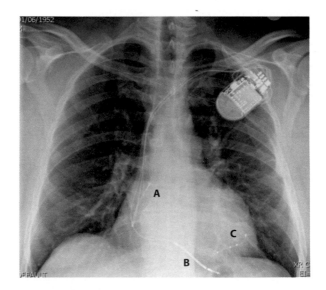

**Figure 5.3** Image of a CRT-D device. Note the three leads (A in right atrial appendage, B in right ventricle and C in left ventricle through the coronary sinus). Note the thickened end of lead B acting as the second point of reference for defibrillation along with the device box.

Cardiology and the cardiovascular system

The table below is reproduced from the NICE guidelines with permissions. It summarizes the indications for these devices.

| QRS INTERVAL | NYHA CLASS | | | |
|---|---|---|---|---|
| | I | II | III | IV |
| <120 milliseconds | ICD if there is a high risk of sudden cardiac death | | | ICD and CRT not clinically Indicated |
| 120–149 milliseconds without LBBB | ICD | ICD | ICD | CRT–P |
| 120–149 milliseconds with LBBB | ICD | CRT–D | CRT–P or CRT–D | CRT–P |
| ≥150 milliseconds with or without LBBB | CRT–D | CRT–D | CRT–P or CRT–D | CRT–P |

LBBB, left bundle branch block; NYHA, New York Heart Association

> **MICRO-reference**
> National Institute for Health and Care Excellence. Implantable cardioverter defibrillators and cardiac resynchronisation therapy for arrhythmias and heart failure (review of TA95 and TA120). London: National Institute for Health and Care Excellence, 2014.

# 5.6 SURGERY FOR HEART FAILURE

## VALVE SURGERY

- Surgery may be appropriate in heart failure due to a valvular aetiology, e.g. aortic valve replacement in severe aortic stenosis.
- Recent advances in percutaneous technologies have made valve interventions accessible even in those not fit for open surgery, e.g. transcatheter aortic valve implantation (TAVI).

## CABG

- Data from a recent trial (STICH, Surgical Treatment for Ischaemic Heart Failure) of 1212 patients with ischaemic cardiomyopathy has suggested that the addition of CABG to medical therapy has no survival advantage except in severe, multivessel, symptomatic angina.

## CARDIAC TRANSPLANTATION

- Cardiac transplantation remains the gold standard therapy for end-stage heart failure resistant to medical therapy.

Cardiology and the cardiovascular system

- Five-year survival is currently upwards of 70%.
- Indications for transplantation:
  - A willingness and ability to withstand the physical and emotional demands of waiting on the transplant list, the procedure and follow-up
  - Objective evidence of limitation (e.g. reduced peak oxygen consumption on cardiopulmonary exercise testing)
  - Patients dependent on intravenous inotropes and mechanical circulatory support

## Contraindications to transplantation:

- Persistent alcohol or drug abuse
- Inadequate control of mental illness
- Treated cancer with remission but less than 5-year follow-up
- Systemic disease with evidence of multi-organ involvement
- Uncontrolled infection
- Severe renal failure
- Fixed high pulmonary vascular resistance
- Recent thromboembolism
- Current gastrointestinal tract ulceration
- Significant hepatic impairment
- Any other medical conditions with a poor prognosis

---

**MICRO-print**
Complications of immunosuppression include:

- Infection
- Hypertension
- Renal failure
- Malignancy

---

## LEFT VENTRICULAR ASSIST DEVICES (LVAD)

- Utilized due to a lack of donor hearts.
- LVADs are pumps which assist the function of the heart.
- LVADs are showing promise as a bridge to transplantation prolonging the lives of those who would otherwise die on the waiting list.
- A new role for LVADs is the support of those with an acute but potentially reversible cause of their heart failure (e.g. post-viral).

---

**MICRO-print**
Complications of LVADs include:

- Increased risk of thromboembolism (need for anti-coagulation)
- Increased risk of infection

---

# 5.7 ADDITIONAL MANAGEMENT

## SMOKING

- Patients with CHF are strongly advised to stop smoking:
  - Increases the risk of cardiovascular disease
  - Reduces cardiac output
  - Reduces lung function and capacity
  - Vasoconstrictive effects

## ALCOHOL

- Reduced alcohol consumption should be encouraged where alcohol relates to the aetiology of the heart failure.
- Alcohol is a myocardial depressant and should be consumed in moderation.

## DIET

- A low salt, low fat, healthy diet should be pursued.
- Weight loss should be encouraged if appropriate.
- In later stages cardiac cachexia is a problem and a poor prognostic feature.

---

### MICRO-facts

**In cardiac cachexia**: there are atrophic changes in the muscles due to metabolic changes, hypo-perfusion and disuse (reduced exercise capacity due to dyspnoea and fatigue). Weight loss is also a result of low appetite, malabsorption and increased metabolic demands.

---

## EXERCISE

- Exercise improves functional capacity and enhances vagal tone.
- Recommend a supervised exercise rehabilitation programme for those with stable disease.

## VACCINATION

- This is important as infection is a significant cause of acute exacerbation.
- A yearly influenza vaccination should be offered.
- A single pneumococcal vaccination should be offered.

## SEXUAL ACTIVITY

- Should be discussed if the patient has concerns.
- Many medications for CHF such as beta-blockers may lead to impotence, therefore the risks and benefits of such therapies should be discussed as appropriate.

Cardiology and the cardiovascular system

## AIR TRAVEL AND DRIVING

- Patients should be made aware that they may be limited in their travel, and this will be dependent on their clinical condition.

> **MICRO-references**
> - The DVLA has specific guidance for patients with heart failure, defibrillators and pacemakers with regards to driving (https://www.gov.uk/health-conditions-and-driving).
> - The civil aviation authority has issued guidance relating to heart failure and air travel (https://www.caa.co.uk/default.aspx/default.aspx?catid=2497&pagetype=90).

# 6 The myocardium

## 6.1 STRUCTURE AND FUNCTION

*Contents:* composed of specialized striated muscle fibres and makes up the bulk of the heart.

*Function:* the myocardium provides the coordinated contractile power to circulate blood.

*Layers:* the myocardium has a smooth surface adjoining the pericardium and a trabeculated surface underlying the endocardium.

It is capable of responding (remodelling) in reaction to altered demands, either physiological or pathological:

- Pressure hypertrophy (the LV has the thickest myocardium and the largest diameter fibres due to the higher pressures).
- Volume dilatation.
- **Hibernation:** myocardium demonstrates altered contractility in response to an insult such as acute myocardial ischaemia; however, this change is potentially reversible over time and with revascularization.

## 6.2 MYOCARDITIS

- Myocarditis describes inflammation of the myocardial tissue.
- It most commonly occurs as part of a generalized viral infection.
- Often associated with pericarditis (myo-pericarditis).
- It is an important component of acute rheumatic fever.

---

**MICRO-print**
Up to 10% of patients with AIDS show cardiac involvement. This may be myocarditis, pericarditis or dilated cardiomyopathy. This may be due to direct effects of the HIV virus or secondary infections.

---

## PATHOLOGY

- Myocardial damage occurs via three mechanisms:
    - Direct invasion of the myocardium
    - Toxin production
    - Immunologically mediated damage

## CAUSES

### Infective

- Viral:
    - Coxsackie B
    - Cytomegalovirus
    - Epstein–Barr virus
    - HIV
- Bacterial:
    - Brucella
    - Diphtheria
    - Staphylococcal or streptococcal (especially pneumococci)
- Fungal
- Protozoa:
    - *Trypanosoma cruzi* is common in South America

### Non-infective

- Toxicity:
    - Heavy metals
    - Drugs:
        - Cyclophosphamide
        - Anthracyclines
- Response to external agents:
    - Radiation
- Autoimmune:
    - Rheumatological: rheumatoid arthritis, systemic lupus erythematosus, sarcoidosis, scleroderma
    - Endocrine: diabetes mellitus, thyroiditis, thyrotoxicosis
    - Neurological: polymyositis, myasthenia gravis

## SIGNS AND SYMPTOMS

- Features vary greatly from subclinical and asymptomatic to fulminant failure:
    - Chest pain is common and is usually due to pericarditis.
    - Tachycardia out of proportion to patient's sepsis or failure:
        - May be bradycardic in diphtheria due to heart block
    - Breathlessness and other signs of left and right heart failure.

INVESTIGATIONS

| Laboratory tests | CRP, ESR | May be raised in inflammatory conditions |
|---|---|---|
| | Troponin | May be raised in myocarditis |
| | Viral titres | |
| ECG | Sinus tachycardia<br>ST/T wave changes especially concave upwards ST elevation<br>T wave inversion<br>Less commonly conduction defects may occur | |
| Echocardiogram | To assess LV dysfunction | |
| Biopsy | Characteristically shows inflammatory cell infiltrates | |

## MICRO-facts

The pericardium is electrically silent, so when ECG changes occur there is always underlying myocardial involvement – known as myo-pericarditis.

MANAGEMENT

- Management is largely supportive.
- Manage heart failure and arrhythmia.
- No specific treatment for viral causes.
- May be a role for corticosteroids in progressive disease.

# 6.3 CARDIOMYOPATHIES

- The cardiomyopathies describe diseases of the heart muscle.
- Can be defined as:
    - **Primary cardiomyopathy:** disease confined to the muscle of the heart and not due to any underlying disease process.
    - **Secondary cardiomyopathy:** disease arising as part of another disease process (sometimes known as specific heart muscle disease – the pattern of muscle involvement may be similar to the primary cardiomyopathies).

## CAUSES OF SECONDARY CARDIOMYOPATHY

- Ischaemic
- Valvular
- Hypertensive
- Nutritional, e.g. thiamine deficiency
- Alcohol
- Peripartum
- Connective tissue diseases
- Substance deposition:
  - Amyloidosis
  - Sarcoidosis
  - Haemachromatosis
- Neuromuscular disease
- Glycogen storage diseases

## HYPERTROPHIC CARDIOMYOPATHY

- Hypertrophic cardiomyopathy describes hypertrophy of the ventricles in the absence of any other cause such as aortic stenosis or hypertension.
- Increased wall stiffness impairs ventricular filling:
  - The result is increased end-diastolic pressure and pulmonary congestion.

### PATHOGENESIS

- Hypertrophy of the myocardium is characteristically heterogeneous (see Figures 6.1 and 6.2).
- It is often most marked at the septum:
  - This may obstruct the left ventricular outflow tract.
  - The obstruction worsens with increased force of contraction.

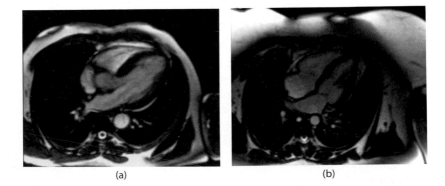

(a)                                                         (b)

**Figure 6.1** Cardiac MRI axial view: (a) ventricular hypertrophy in this patient with hypertrophic cardiomyopathy is demonstrable when compared to (b) normal ventricular wall.

Cardiology and the cardiovascular system

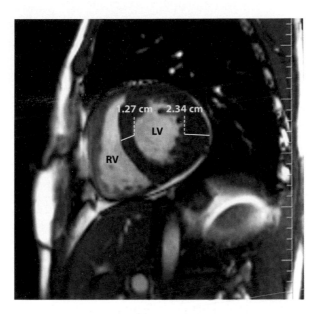

**Figure 6.2** Short axis view of hypertrophic cardiomyopathy. Short axis cine view of the heart on cardiac MRI showing asymmetrical hypertrophy of the lateral wall in a patient with hypertrophic cardiomyopathy.

- The anterolateral wall is often affected more than the posterior wall.
- The LV is more affected than the RV.
- Isolated apical hypertrophy is more common in Japan.
- Occasionally, symmetrical hypertrophy is seen.
- Histologically myocardial fibre disarray, hypertrophy and interstitial fibrosis may be seen.

### GENETICS

- A number of genes on several chromosomes have been identified:
  - Autosomal-dominant inheritance is present in up to 50% of cases.
- Even with specific defects, there is a large difference in expression between patients.
- Familial screening is important and a large number of cases are now identified this way.

---

**MICRO-print**
Increasingly, sportsmen and women are screened for the possibility of hypertrophic cardiomyopathy following a number of high profile deaths in young athletes. Initial assessment is by ECG with or without echocardiography.

Cardiology and the cardiovascular system

## FEATURES

- Symptoms normally of pulmonary congestion and dyspnoea
- Signs include:
    - Jerky pulse
    - Atrial fibrillation is common
    - Prominent 'a' wave in JVP waveform
    - Double apex beat
    - S3 and S4
    - Late ejection systolic murmur over the aortic area
    - Often a mitral regurgitant murmur

## INVESTIGATIONS

| ECG | May show LVH with deep S waves in septal hypertrophy<br>ST segment and T wave abnormalities<br>P wave may reflect atrial enlargement (see Chapter 12, P wave section) |
|---|---|
| Echocardiogram | Can show non-concentric hypertrophy<br>Asymmetrical hypertrophy of the septum<br>Obliteration of the ventricular cavity during systole<br>Systolic anterior motion of the mitral valve<br>Mitral regurgitation |
| MRI | Shows LV hypertrophy<br>Evidence of outflow obstruction<br>Demonstrates myocardial fibrosis |
| Angiography | Demonstrates a small cavity<br>Narrowing of the outflow tract<br>Mitral regurgitation |

## MANAGEMENT

- The mainstay of treatment is medical:
    - Beta-blockers and rate-limiting calcium channel antagonists improve ventricular filling by prolonging diastole.
    - Arrythmias are common (especially atrial fibrillation) and may necessitate beta-blockade:
        - Anti-arrhythmic drugs such as amiodarone may be employed, although the evidence base is weak.
- Alcohol septal ablation can be used percutaneously:
    - Arteries supplying the septum are isolated and alcohol introduced to induce a local infarction.

- Surgery may be necessary in some cases:
  - Myocardium is removed surgically to widen the outflow tract.
  - Conduction defects are common.
- Dual chamber pacing can improve symptoms when septal reduction is contraindicated but this is rarely used now (LBBB is induced to desynchronize the septum and posterior wall which reduces outflow obstruction).
- Implantable cardio-defibrillators are indicated in those at high risk of sudden death.

## DILATED CARDIOMYOPATHY

- Dilated cardiomyopathy is the final manifestation of a number of disease processes leading to ventricular dilatation (see Figure 6.3).
- May be familial although sporadic cases are more common.

### CAUSES

- Treatable causes must be excluded to reach a diagnosis:
  - Coronary disease
  - Valvular disease
  - Congenital disease
- Common causes are:
  - Alcohol
  - Myocarditis
  - Chemotherapy
  - Haemachromatosis
  - Thyrotoxicosis
  - Thiamine deficiency

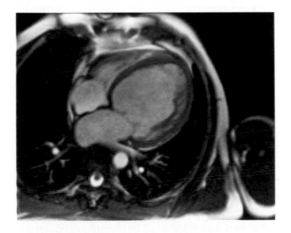

**Figure 6.3** Cardiac MRI axial view showing dilated cardiomyopathy.

> ## MICRO-facts
> The most common cause of dilated cardiomyopathy in the Western world is alcohol excess. Damage may occur due to the toxicity of alcohol and associated vitamin deficiencies. Cessation of drinking and treatment of vitamin deficiency can halt progression.

### FEATURES

- Presents with symptoms of heart failure.
- Atrial fibrillation is common due to LA enlargement.
- S3 and S4 are common.
- Mitral and tricuspid regurgitant murmurs frequently occur.

### INVESTIGATIONS

| ECG | Shows arrhythmias and ST segment and T wave abnormality<br>Absence of Q waves is important in ruling out previous infarction as a cause for symptoms |
|---|---|
| CXR | Cardiomegaly and increased pulmonary vascular congestion |
| Echo | Dilated ventricles<br>Poor contractile function<br>Global impairment (infarction gives regional impairment)<br>May show valvular regurgitation due to, e.g. stretch of the AV valve annulus |
| MRI | Ventricular dilatation and changes in wall thickness |
| Angiography | May exclude coronary artery disease<br>Forms part of the work-up towards a cardiac transplant |
| Biopsy | Commonly shows end-stage fibrosis |

### MANAGEMENT

- Identifiable causes should be treated.
- Treatment focuses on relief of heart failure:
  - ACE inhibitors
  - Beta-blockers
  - Spironolactone
  - Diuretics for symptomatic relief
- Anti-coagulation may be indicated as frequently atrial arrhythmias coexist.
- Cardiac resynchronization may benefit a small number of patients.
- In end-stage disease, cardiac transplantation may become necessary.

> **MICRO-print**
> **Takotsubo cardiomyopathy** (stress-related) is a condition character-
> ized by transient LV apical ballooning seen on echocardiography.
> Presents with chest pain associated with emotional stress and
> resembles an acute coronary syndrome. Ischaemic ECG changes and
> raised cardiac enzymes are seen but coronary angiography is normal.
> Changes seen on echocardiography usually return to normal within
> weeks.
>
> **Peripartum cardiomyopathy** is an uncommon cardiomyopathy of
> unknown aetiology that may be progressive and severe. The diag-
> nosis is made when an ejection fraction of less than 45% develops
> either in the last month of pregnancy or within 5 months of partum in
> the absence of any other cause of heart failure. Outcomes for peri-
> partum cardiomyopathy have improved with advances in pharmaco-
> logical and device treatments, with estimated 5-year survival rates
> as high as 90–95%.

## RESTRICTIVE AND INFILTRATIVE CARDIOMYOPATHY

- Restrictive cardiomyopathy leads to myocardial stiffness and a non-
  compliant ventricle:
    - Leads to poor ventricular filling and diastolic dysfunction.
    - Systolic function may be maintained.

### CAUSES

- The most common causes are:
    - Haemachromatosis
    - Sarcoidosis
    - Amyloidosis
    - Carcinoid syndrome
    - Glycogen storage diseases
    - Endomyocardial fibrosis

### SIGNS AND SYMPTOMS

- Normally presents with predominantly right-sided heart failure:
    - Peripheral oedema
    - Raised JVP:
        - Rapid 'x' and 'y' descents
    - Hepatomegaly
- Loud S3 and S4

Cardiology and the cardiovascular system

## INVESTIGATIONS

| Laboratory investigations | May show a cause such as sarcoidosis or amyloidosis |
|---|---|
| ECG | Subendocardial fibrosis may lead to conduction defects<br>May show low voltages in amyloidosis |
| Echocardiography | Abnormal tissue characteristics (infiltration) may be found although there may be no hypertrophy or dilatation<br>Often apparent normal systolic function<br>Diastolic dysfunction is seen<br>There may be bi-atrial enlargement |
| MRI | Increasingly used to assist diagnosis |

## MANAGEMENT

- No specific therapies and largely supportive.
- Treating the causative disease may be effective.
- Disease is commonly progressive.

## ARRHYTHMOGENIC RIGHT VENTRICULAR DYSPLASIA (ARVD)

- Also known as arrhythmogenic right ventricular cardiomyopathy.
- This is a rare cardiomyopathy often with autosomal-dominant inheritance.
- Affects predominantly the RV but may involve both.

## SYMPTOMS

- Often presents with features of arrhythmia:
  - Palpitations
  - Dizziness
  - Syncope
- Elements of heart failure may be apparent.

## INVESTIGATIONS

| ECG | Diagnosis of ARVD should be considered in patients with VT with a LBBB (right ventricular origin)<br>Epsilon waves (small terminal upward deflection in the QRS complex) in a signal-averaged ECG |
|---|---|

*Continued*

| Echocardiography | Frequently normal but may show RV enlargement |
|---|---|
| **Biopsy** | Fatty infiltration is characteristic but may be patchy |
| **MRI** | Gold standard for diagnosis<br>Can show infiltration, wall thinning or abnormal contraction |

MANAGEMENT

- Management focuses on controlling arrhythmias.
- Beta-blockers and particularly sotalol are useful.
- There is a risk of sudden arrhythmic death and an ICD may be indicated.

---

**MICRO-case**

A 55-year-old man with a history of alcohol excess presented to his GP with breathlessness on exertion. On examination, it was noted that he had an irregularly irregular pulse at 70 bpm, a normal respiratory rate, his chest was clear and he had normal oxygen saturations. There was pedal oedema and a mildly raised JVP. The GP arranged blood tests to measure FBC, LFT, U&E, TFT and serum natriuretic peptides (BNP/NTproBNP). A plain chest radiograph was organised, as was an ECG that revealed atrial fibrillation with a slow ventricular response. Based on the patient preference and CHADSVASc and HASBLED scores, it was decided to anti-coagulate him with warfarin and to treat him with rate-controlling bisoprolol (see p. 176). An urgent echocardiogram demonstrated dilatation of all four chambers with LV systolic dysfunction. The GP suspected alcohol-induced dilated cardiomyopathy and referred him to a cardiologist for further management. He was advised to reduce his alcohol intake and was given thiamine and vitamin B replacement to prevent Wernicke's encephalopathy. He was commenced on an ACE inhibitor in addition to his beta-blockade to treat his heart failure.

**Points to consider:**

- Cardiomyopathies are a significant cause of arrhythmias.
- Dilated cardiomyopathy may be secondary to chronic and excessive alcohol abuse.
- In patients with newly diagnosed AF, it is important to enquire about systemic symptoms and alcohol history, and to organize an echocardiogram, electrolytes and thyroid function tests.

Cardiology and the cardiovascular system

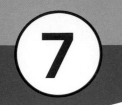

# Pericardial disease

## 7.1 THE PERICARDIAL SAC

*Contents:* completely encompasses all cardiac chambers aside from a portion of the LA

*Function:* acts as a protective and lubricating covering around the heart

*Layers:* located within the mediastinum, the pericardium is made up of two layers

- **Fibrous** outer layer tethered to the central tendon of the diaphragm
- **Serous** inner layer made of two layers between which there is a closed pericardial cavity, a space containing 15–50 ml of lubricating pericardial fluid:
  - **Parietal pericardium** fused with the fibrous outer layer
  - **Visceral pericardium** fused with the epicardium

## 7.2 ACUTE PERICARDITIS

### Symptoms

- Sharp, central chest pain that radiates to the scapular ridge
- Worsened by lying, movement and inspiration
- Relieved by leaning forward
- Systemic symptoms (fever, chills)

### Signs

- Pyrexia
- Tachypnoea
- Tachycardia
- Pericardial friction rub

> **MICRO-facts**
>
> Pericardial friction rubs are pathognomonic but not always present. Listen on the left lower sternal edge with the patient leaning forward. It sounds scratchy and occurs in both systole and diastole.

## AETIOLOGY

Inflammation of the pericardium can be divided into infective and non-infective:

- **Infective:**
  - Viral
  - Bacterial
  - Fungal
- **Non-infective:**
  - Post-infarction
  - Trauma
  - Autoimmune:
    - Dressler's syndrome (post-infarction antibody formation)
    - Rheumatoid
    - Vasculitis
    - Systemic lupus erythematosus
    - Scleroderma
  - Uraemic
  - Iatrogenic:
    - Post-thoracic surgery
    - Post-resuscitation
    - Tetracycline-induced
  - Neoplastic:
    - Primary or metastatic
    - Paraneoplastic
    - Secondary to radiation therapy

## INVESTIGATIONS

| Laboratory tests | CRP, ESR<br>Troponin<br>Viral titres<br>Autoimmune<br>  profile | Raised in inflammatory aetiology<br>May be raised due to associated<br>  myocarditis<br>If Troponin negative can exclude<br>  infarction |
|---|---|---|
| ECG | | Saddle-shaped concave upwards ST elevation across<br>  the ECG (see Figure 7.1)<br>Changes are not confined to a single arterial territory |
| CXR | | May show an effusion or signs of tuberculosis |
| Echo | | Mandatory in order to identify the presence of<br>  an effusion |

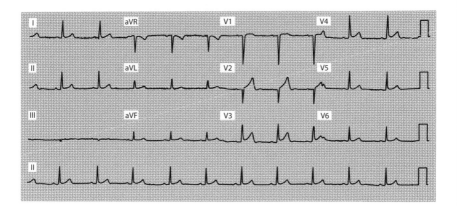

**Figure 7.1** Image ECG of pericarditis with widespread saddle-shaped ST segment elevation.

### TREATMENT

- **NSAIDs** (aspirin, indomethacin, ibuprofen) reduce pain and inflammation.
- **Colchicine** reduces relapse.
- **Corticosteroids** for pericarditis of autoimmune, connective tissue or uraemic aetiology.

### COMPLICATIONS

- Pericardial effusion and cardiac tamponade
- Chronic pericarditis (pericarditis persisting beyond 6 months)
- Constrictive pericarditis – may require pericardiectomy if severe
- Recurrent pericarditis (not always associated with other autoimmune diseases)

## 7.3 PERICARDIAL EFFUSION AND CARDIAC TAMPONADE

*Pericardial effusion* is the presence of excess fluid between the parietal and visceral pericardium.

*Cardiac tamponade* is a pericardial effusion that has resulted in haemodynamic compromise.

**Physiology:** Transformation of an effusion into a tamponade is dependent not just on volume, but also on the rate of development. Rapidly developing effusions do not allow the heart to accommodate and therefore may compromise cardiac output.

Cardiology and the cardiovascular system

**AETIOLOGY**

- Often secondary to pericarditis
- Can be divided into:
  - Transudates (lower protein content):
    - Heart failure
    - Renal failure
    - Liver failure
    - Myxoedema
  - Exudates (higher protein content):
    - Infection
    - Malignancy
    - Autoimmune
  - Pyopericardium (pus)
  - Haemopericardium (blood):
    - Trauma
    - Malignancy

---

## MICRO-facts

Haemopericardium is blood in the pericardium and can result from cardiac rupture, cardiac surgery, tuberculosis and neoplastic invasion.

---

**SYMPTOMS**

- Chest pain relieved by leaning forward
- Palpitations
- Pressure on surrounding structures:
  - Breathlessness (lung)
  - Hiccups (phrenic nerve)
  - Nausea

---

**MICRO-print**

*Post-cardiotomy syndrome* occurs weeks after cardiac surgery and is due to the development of autoantibodies against damaged cardiac tissue. It presents as a flu-like illness, petechiae on the skin and pericarditis with effusion. The condition responds to immunosuppression/steroids.

## SIGNS

Pericardial effusions may be associated with no signs, but cardiac tamponade results in signs through a threefold mechanism:
- Fluid and pressure effects on the heart and surrounding structures:
  - Muffled heart sounds
  - Impalpable apex beat
  - Dyspnoea
  - Pulsus paradoxus
  - Ewart's sign: dullness to percussion and bronchial breathing at the inferior angle of the left scapula due to compression of the left lower lung lobe by pericardial fluid
- Back pressure:
  - Kussmaul's sign
  - Raised JVP with loss of 'y' descent
- Inability to maintain a cardiac output leads to signs of shock.
  If left untreated, tamponade leads to death.

---

### MICRO-print

**Pulsus paradoxus** refers to a drop of >10 mmHg in BP during inspiration, clinically resulting in some heartbeats that are auscultated but cannot be felt at the radial pulse (this is the 'paradox' of the pulse). This is not a paradoxical phenomenon at all, but an exaggeration of the normal response. In normal physiology, inspiration decreases intrathoracic pressure, pooling venous blood in the right-heart chambers and pulmonary circulation. This in turn decreases LV preload and cardiac output (Frank–Starling mechanism) and systolic BP drops by <10 mmHg. In cardiac tamponade, the mechanism producing pulsus paradoxus is complex. In essence, the fluid-filled pericardial sac prevents the blood-filled RV from expanding outwards and causes the septum to deviate towards the LV, further reducing filling and cardiac output. During expiration, the presence of a less-filled RV means the LV has space to fill and increase cardiac output. This phenomenon is known as *ventricular interdependence*.

Pulsus paradoxus may also be observed in severe asthma attacks or severe COPD.

**Kussmaul's sign** is a rise in JVP with inspiration instead of a fall as would be expected due to increased venous return to the heart (true paradox). This is suggestive of right-heart diastolic dysfunction due to cardiac tamponade, constrictive pericarditis or restrictive cardiomyopathy.

## MICRO-facts

**Beck's triad:** Hypotension + raised JVP + muffled heart sounds caused by cardiac tamponade.

### INVESTIGATIONS

| | |
|---|---|
| **ECG** | Low-voltage complexes (common)<br>Electrical alternans: changing QRS complex axis or amplitude as the heart is oscillating in the pericardial fluid (uncommon) |
| **CXR** | Globular heart (see Figure 7.2) |
| **Echocardiogram** | Extent of an effusion and any evidence of myocardial rupture may be assessed<br>Criteria for tamponade may be assessed |
| **Pericardiocentesis** | Look for<br>• Evidence to suggest an exudative process:<br>  • Raised effusion: serum LDH<br>  • Raised effusion: serum protein<br>• Viral PCR<br>• Microscopy and cell count<br>• Culture and gram-staining<br>• Cytology for malignant cells |

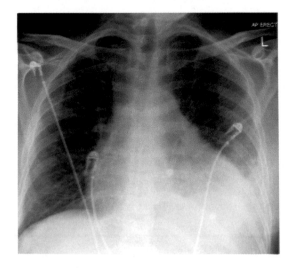

Figure 7.2 Globular heart in cardiac tamponade.

TREATMENT

- Cardiac tamponade is a *medical emergency*: use ABCDE and supportive therapies:
  - Oxygen (avoid CPAP as this further reduces venous return)
  - Fluids and cardiac inotropic drugs in case of shock
  - Morphine for pain and anxiety
- Remove excess fluid:
  - Emergency subxiphoid percutaneous drainage
  - Echocardiogram-guided pericardiocentesis
- Prevent recurrence (frequent, recurrence is 13–50% for malignant effusions):
  - *Non-surgical:*
    - Percutaneous balloon pericardiotomy
    - Intrapericardial administration of sclerosing agents binds the two layers of pericardium together and obliterates the potential space
  - *Surgical:*
    - Pleuro-pericardial window formation (creation of a fistula between the pericardial and pleural space)
    - Pericardio-peritoneal shunt

# 7.4 CONSTRICTIVE PERICARDITIS

- May occur secondary to any form of chronic pericarditis (lasting over 3 months)
- Scar-like fibrosis and adhesions within the pericardium
- Most commonly the aetiology is:
  - Idiopathic
  - Post-cardiac surgery
  - Radiation to the mediastinum
  - Connective tissue disorder
  - Tuberculous pericarditis
  - Bacterial pericarditis
  - Haemorrhagic pericarditis

The fibrocalcific shell prevents chamber filling, resulting in a predominantly biventricular diastolic dysfunction.

PRESENTATION

- Right heart failure symptoms and signs predominate.
- Left heart failure symptoms may also be present.
- Presence of a pulsus paradoxus is uncommon, but Kussmaul's sign may be present.
- Hepatomegaly and ascites.

Cardiology and the cardiovascular system

## INVESTIGATIONS

| ECG | Diffuse low-voltage complexes<br>Non-specific ST segment and T wave changes<br>Atrial fibrillation |
|---|---|
| CXR | Pericardial calcification may be present but does not imply physiologically significant disease |
| Echo | Preserved ventricular systolic function<br>Small ventricles<br>Dilated atria<br>Excess movement of interventricular septum |
| CT/MRI | Best non-invasive measure of pericardial thickness (thickness ≥4 mm) |
| Cardiac catheterization | Both right-sided and left-sided catheterization should be performed with simultaneous recording of intracardiac pressures<br>Diastolic pressures may be equal in all four chambers |

## TREATMENT

- **Medical management** is palliative:
  - Diuretics and venodilators for right-sided heart failure
- **Surgical management** can be curative:
  - Surgical resection of the pericardium
  - Best performed early as duration of symptoms correlates with poor outcome post-surgery
- Poor prognostic indicators:
  - Increasing age
  - Long-standing condition
  - Post-radiation aetiology
  - LV systolic dysfunction

---

**MICRO-print**

**Cardiac tamponade versus constrictive pericarditis**

Both these conditions may present with diastolic dysfunction. Differentiation is facilitated by the use of echocardiograms outlining significant pericardial effusions in cardiac tamponade. Pulsus paradoxus is present usually in tamponade but not in constrictive pericarditis: the fibrocalcific shell acts as a divider between intrathoracic and intrapericardial pressures. This means that the normal fall in

*continued...*

*continued...*

intrathoracic pressure with inspiration is not transmitted to the cardiac chambers. Venous return and RV filling are therefore affected less by inspiration, and so a decrease in LV filling and cardiac output on inspiration (pulsus paradoxus) may not be present.

### Constrictive pericarditis versus restrictive cardiomyopathy

Both conditions result in diastolic dysfunction of the heart with right-heart failure. Differentiation is essential as constriction may be treated surgically. The diagnosis may be aided by measuring pericardial thickening but a normal thickness cannot exclude constrictive pericarditis. An endomyocardial biopsy is not routine but it can diagnose an infiltrative restrictive cardiomyopathy. Moreover, separation of the intrathoracic and intrapericardial pressures is present in constrictive pericarditis but not in restrictive cardiomyopathy. Therefore, haemodynamic studies comprising right-heart and left-heart catheterization with assessment of the effect of the respiratory cycle can aid the diagnosis.

### MICRO-case

A 60-year-old man presented to the ED with sudden onset of sharp central chest pain, worse on inspiration and relieved by leaning forward. He explained to the attending doctor that he was apprehensive, as he had had a severe chest pain 3 weeks ago that he had ignored as it had eventually settled. His relatives persuaded him to attend the department 48 hours later and the diagnosis of anterior STEMI was made resulting in late reperfusion angioplasty. On examination, he had normal blood pressure, pulse, heart sounds and air entry. On the ECG, there was generalized ST segment elevation in all leads with no ST depression. His blood tests revealed a moderate troponin level and raised CRP and ESR. Based on the history, ECG changes, serial troponin levels and elevated inflammatory markers, a provisional diagnosis of Dressler's syndrome was made and he was given a short course of colchicine. A cardiology opinion was obtained to consider and exclude the important differential diagnosis of stent thrombosis in a patient with chest pain and recent angioplasty. An inpatient chest radiograph revealed bibasal small pleural effusions and an echocardiogram revealed a small pericardial effusion. The pain resolved and he was discharged with cardiology follow-up.

### Points to consider:

- In pericarditis, ST changes are generalized and not limited to a single coronary vessel territory.
- Dressler's syndrome is due to the development of antibodies to damaged myocardium.
- The condition is becoming less common with the advent of early reperfusion therapy by thrombolysis and primary PCI.

Cardiology and the cardiovascular system

# 8 The cardiac valves

## 8.1 STRUCTURE OF VALVES

Common features shared by all four valves:
- Three layers of connective tissue with an overlying endothelial layer
- Avascular valve leaflets that overlap when closed
- Open and close in response to pressure changes across the valve

> **MICRO-facts**
>
> The meeting of two opposing valve leaflets at the point of their insertion is known as the **commissure**.

### FUNCTION

- Atrioventricular valves:
  - Close in systole
  - Open in diastole
  - Closure forms the first heart sound
- Semilunar valves:
  - Open in systole
  - Close in diastole
  - Closure forms the second heart sound

### ATRIOVENTRICULAR VALVES (MITRAL AND TRICUSPID)

- The tricuspid valve has three leaflets.
- The mitral valve has two leaflets.
- Valve leaflets are inserted into a fibrous ring in the atrioventricular wall (annulus).
- The subvalvular apparatus consisting of the chordae tendinae and papillary muscles prevents the AV valves prolapsing into the atria when ventricular pressure increases:
  - **Chordae tendinae** connect the cusp to the papillary muscles.
  - **Papillary muscles** connect the chordae tendinae to the ventricular wall.

## SEMILUNAR VALVES (AORTIC AND PULMONARY)

- Aortic and pulmonary valves with three equally spaced commissures.
- Above, the cusps insert into a fibrous sleeve attached into the vessel.
- Below, the cusps are attached into the ventricular outflow tract.
- More similar in structure to valves in the veins than the AV valves.
- The coronary artery sinuses lie just above the aortic valve and fill in diastole.

# 8.2 INFECTIVE ENDOCARDITIS

- This is an uncommon condition with significant mortality.
- It is an infection of the endocardium, particularly affecting the valve leaflets and the subvalvular apparatus.

## TYPES OF ENDOCARDITIS

### Native valve endocarditis

- The majority of cases occur in patients with a predisposing lesion.
- Formerly, most commonly due to rheumatic heart disease but now other pathologies predominate.
- Can present in two ways:
  - **Acute native valve endocarditis:**
    - More likely to affect normal valves
    - Aggressive course
  - **Subacute native valve endocarditis:**
    - More likely to affect abnormal valves
    - Less aggressive course over weeks or months

### Endocarditis in intravenous drug users (IVDU)

- Endocarditis without underlying valve pathology is common in IVDUs.
- Normally affects the tricuspid valve (approximately 80%).
  - Mitral and aortic valves may also be affected.
  - Pulmonary valve rarely affected.
- In contrast to left-sided endocarditis, multiple septic emboli may dislodge from the tricuspid valvular vegetations and form pulmonary emboli presenting with symptoms of pneumonia.

### Prosthetic valve endocarditis

- Can be divided into early (within the first 60 days of implantation) and late endocarditis.
- Early infection is often due to perioperative contamination:
  - Majority of cases are due to staphylococcal infection.
  - Sources include peripheral and central access lines and urinary catheters.
- Late infection resembles native valve endocarditis.

## AETIOLOGY

- *Streptococci:*
  - Account for 50–80% of cases.
  - *Viridans* group *streptococci* form the normal flora of the pharynx and upper respiratory tract – dental surgery, pharyngeal surgery and even tooth cleaning can cause bacteraemia and infection.
  - *S. bovis* and *S. faecalis* colonize the gastrointestinal tract and may give rise to endocarditis in the presence of gastrointestinal pathology.
- *Staphylococci:*
  - *S. aureus* and *S. epidermidis* are skin commensals and account for an increasing proportion of infective endocarditis.
  - *S. aureus* is the most common pathogen causing endocarditis in IVDU.
  - *S. epidermidis* is responsible for a large proportion of prosthetic valve endocarditis with infected cannulae and central lines being a possible source.
- *Enterococci:*
  - Account for a minority of cases
  - Normally bowel flora with low infectivity
- HACEK organisms – blood cultures may be negative as these organisms require special growth media:
  - *Haemophilus parainfluenza* and *Haemophilus aphrophilus*
  - *Actinobacillus actinomycetemcomitans*
  - *Cardiobacterium hominis*
  - *Eikenella* species
  - *Kingella* species
- Others (rare):
  - *Candida*
  - *Aspergillus*
  - *Histoplasma*
  - *Brucella*
  - *Coxiella burnetii* (Q fever)

## PATHOLOGY

- Endocarditis is thought to occur where a high-pressure jet of blood enters a low-pressure region:
  - Pressure damages the endocardium and creates an area for bacteria to settle.
  - Endocarditis is associated with small ventriculo-septal defects due to the higher pressure across smaller defects.
    - Less commonly associated with atrial septal defects
    - Occurs only rarely in pure mitral stenosis

- Infection leads to vegetation formation that consists of clot and bacteria held together by agglutinating proteins.
- Organisms then invade the valve leaflet and surrounding structures, which may lead to:
  - Erosion or perforation that may progress to valvular incompetence
  - Abscess formation
  - Cardiac conduction defects if in the septal area
  - Rupture of the sinus of Valsalva or aneurysm formation if in the aortic area

---

## MICRO-facts

**Embolization effects:**
- Pulmonary embolization
- Myocardial infarction
- Splenic infarction
- Mesenteric infarction
- Renal infarction
- Stroke

---

### SYMPTOMS

- Fever and night sweats
- Malaise
- Weight loss
- Arthralgia
- Back pain

### SIGNS

- **A new or changing murmur.**
- Finger clubbing and splenomegaly can occur in subacute disease.
- JVP may demonstrate features of tricuspid regurgitation (large 'v' waves).
- Acute heart failure if valvular incompetence occurs.
- Immune complex deposition manifesting as:
  - Petechiae and splinter haemorrhages in nail beds
  - Janeway lesions – painless erythematous macules on the palms
  - Osler's nodes – tender erythematous nodules on the pulps of the fingers
  - Roth's spots – retinal haemorrhages
  - Microscopic haematuria due to glomerulonephritis

INVESTIGATIONS

| Laboratory tests | FBC | Usually normocytic, normochromic anaemia |
|---|---|---|
| | U&E | Renal failure due to glomerulonephritis |
| | CRP | May be used to monitor disease progression |
| | Blood cultures | Around 85% of cases have positive cultures At least three sets (aerobic and anaerobic bottles) from different sites over 48 hours are required |
| | Urine dipstick | Look for micro-haematuria |
| ECG | | May show conduction defects First-degree heart block may be a sign of aortic root involvement |
| CXR | | May show evidence of heart failure |
| Echocardiography | | Trans-oesophageal echocardiography identifies vegetation better than transthoracic echocardiography (TTE) and is preferable for suspected right-sided lesions (see Figure 8.1) |

DUKE CRITERIA

- The Duke criteria aid diagnosis based on signs and symptoms:
  - Definite infective endocarditis requires one of the following:
    - Two major criteria
    - One major and three minor criteria
    - Five minor criteria

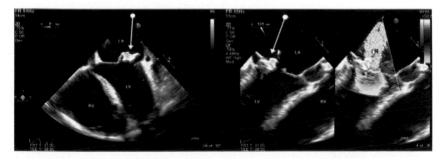

**Figure 8.1** Infective endocarditis with vegetations. Mid-oesophageal four-chamber and three-chamber views of mitral valve leaflets on trans-oesophageal echocardiography. This is showing vegetation on the tip of the anterior mitral valve leaflet (arrows). The anterior mitral valve leaflet is flail and its tip is displaced in the left atrium during systole resulting in torrential mitral regurgitation clearly shown on colour Doppler.

Cardiology and the cardiovascular system

- Possible infective endocarditis is suggested by one of the following:
    - One major and one minor criteria
    - Three minor criteria

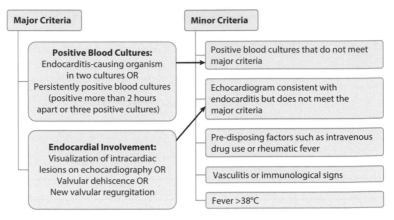

| Major Criteria | Minor Criteria |
|---|---|
| **Positive Blood Cultures:** Endocarditis-causing organism in two cultures OR Persistently positive blood cultures (positive more than 2 hours apart or three positive cultures) | Positive blood cultures that do not meet major criteria |
| | Echocardiogram consistent with endocarditis but does not meet the major criteria |
| **Endocardial Involvement:** Visualization of intracardiac lesions on echocardiography OR Valvular dehiscence OR New valvular regurgitation | Pre-disposing factors such as intravenous drug use or rheumatic fever |
| | Vasculitis or immunological signs |
| | Fever >38°C |

## MANAGEMENT

- Intravenous antibiotics are required following blood cultures:
    - Should be targeted by culture and sensitivity studies.
    - Empirical treatment according to local guidelines may be commenced in culture negative endocarditis.
- Involvement of microbiology service is essential especially in rare causes of endocarditis.
- Treatment needs to continue for an extended course to ensure resolution of the infection.
- Surgery may be indicated in a small number of cases:
    - Is usually delayed to allow antibiotics to control the infection
    - Indications include:
        - Development of congestive heart failure or tissue destruction, e.g. aortic abscess
        - Failure of drug treatment to eradicate sepsis
        - Unusual or multi-resistant organism
        - Large mobile vegetations with risk of embolization

---

## MICRO-facts

In some cases, individuals at risk of endocarditis may require prophylactic antibiotics before high-risk procedures.

---

Cardiology and the cardiovascular system

# 8.3 AETIOLOGY OF VALVE DISEASE

## PRIMARY CAUSES

- Rheumatic heart disease
- Degenerative calcification – calcific aortic stenosis and calcification of the mitral annulus
- Myxomatous degeneration (connective tissue weakening) – affects the mitral valve
- Infective endocarditis
- Congenital – as part of a complex or an isolated defect

## SECONDARY CAUSES

### Cardiac disease

- Ischaemic – acute or chronic regurgitation due to papillary muscle or chordae tendinae dysfunction or altered ventricular wall motility
- Functional – change to the dimensions of the ventricle leading to changes to the valve root

### Systemic disease

- **Connective tissue disease** either inherited (e.g. Marfan's syndrome, Ehlers–Danlos syndrome, osteogenesis imperfecta) or acquired
- **Systemic inflammatory diseases** (e.g. giant cell arteritis, rheumatoid arthritis, ankylosing spondylitis, Reiter's disease, Takayasu's disease, Behçet's syndrome)
- Inborn errors of metabolism
- Carcinoid syndrome
- Systemic amyloidosis or senile cardiac amyloidosis
- Radiation

# 8.4 AORTIC VALVE

## AORTIC VALVE STENOSIS (AS)

- Commonly due to disease of the valve cusps
- May also occur due to narrowing of the outflow tract (subvalvar stenosis) or narrowing of the first part of the aorta (supravalvular stenosis)

### Causes

- **Congenital** stenosis is usually due to a bicuspid valve, which has a tendency to calcify.
- **Rheumatic** stenosis results from cusp fusion and calcification following rheumatic fever.
- **Senile** stenosis results from degeneration and consequent calcium deposition.

Cardiology and the cardiovascular system

## SYMPTOMS

- Classical triad of symptoms: **breathlessness, exertional syncope** and **angina** (AS reduces coronary flow reserve and AS-induced LVH also results in myocardial ischaemia)
- Later symptoms:
  - Orthopnoea and paroxysmal nocturnal dyspnoea from pulmonary congestion
  - Congestive cardiac failure symptoms

## SIGNS

- Slow-rising and reduced amplitude pulse
- Heaving apex that may be displaced downwards as in heart failure

---

**The murmur**

An **ejection systolic (crescendo–decrescendo pattern) murmur is heard over the upper right sternal edge radiating to the carotids.** S2 is soft (as the aortic component becomes quieter with increasing severity, a loud S2 indicates that AS is unlikely) and can be split due to late aortic closure. An ejection click may be present.

---

## INVESTIGATIONS

| ECG | LVH |
|---|---|
| CXR | May show chamber enlargement or pulmonary congestion |
| Echocardiography | Shows thickened valve leaflets with restricted opening<br>May show hypertrophy of the left ventricular walls<br>The severity of the stenosis can be assessed by the valve orifice and the gradient (see Figure 8.2) |

The ACC/AHA criteria for AS severity:

| | MILD | MODERATE | SEVERE | CRITICAL |
|---|---|---|---|---|
| Mean gradient (mmHg) | <20 | 20–40 | >40 | >70 |
| Aortic valve area (cm²) | >1.5 | 1.0–1.5 | <1.0 | <0.6 |
| Jet velocity (m/s) | 2.6–2.9 m/s | 3–4 m/s | >4 m/s | |

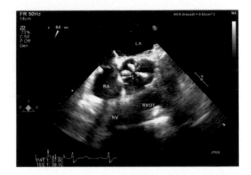

**Figure 8.2** Aortic stenosis. Upper mid-oesophageal view of aortic valve on trans-oesophageal echocardiography. The aortic valve is tri-leaflet and has significant calcium burden. Valve area on planimetry is only 0.65 cm², which is consistent with severe aortic stenosis.

---

**MICRO-references**

Baumgartner H, Hung J, Bermejo J, et al. Echocardiographic assessment of valve stenosis: EAE/ASE recommendations for clinical practice. *European Journal of Echocardiography* 2009; 10(1): 1–25.
ESC/EACTS Guidelines. Guidelines on the management of valvular heart disease. *European Heart Journal* 2012; 33: 2451–2496.

---

TREATMENT

- As is usually slowly progressive with a long asymptomatic period and may require no specific treatment.
- Patients require regular follow-up to assess symptoms and AS severity on TTE.
- Surgery is indicated in severe stenosis that is symptomatic:
    - It is often carried out at the same time as CABG operations.
- Percutaneous valve implants are a new option for patients not fit for open surgery, e.g. transcatheter aortic valve implantation.

---

**MICRO-print**

Heyde's syndrome describes colonic angiodysplasia and bleeding due to aortic stenosis. It is now understood that the aortic stenosis induces a form of von Willebrand's disease. This quickly resolves with resolution of the stenosis. It is thought that the turbulent flow of blood across the valve leads to splitting of the large von Willebrand's molecule.

Cardiology and the cardiovascular system

> ## MICRO-facts
>
> Avoid the use of nitrates in severe aortic stenosis as this may cause venous dilatation and reduce preload, further reducing cardiac output. The use of glyceryl trinitrate spray may cause severe systemic hypotension.

## AORTIC VALVE REGURGITATION (AR)

### CAUSES

- May be due to intrinsic disease of the valve or stretching of the aortic root.

#### Acute regurgitation

- Acute regurgitation is a complication of aortic dissection.
- Infective endocarditis is the other most common cause of acute AR.
- The ventricle has not had time to adapt to the large increase in blood volume resulting in:
  - Decreased stroke volume
  - Tachycardia
  - Pulmonary oedema
  - Cardiogenic shock
- This is an emergency and requires urgent treatment both medically and surgically.

#### Chronic regurgitation

Can be caused by:
- Damage from infective endocarditis
- Rheumatic involvement of the aortic valve leading to thickening of the cusps and fusion of the commissures
- Dilatation of the aortic root from aneurysm of the ascending aorta is seen in:
  - Long-standing poorly controlled hypertension
  - Marfan's syndrome and other connective tissue disease
  - Syphilitic aortitis

### SYMPTOMS

- Dyspnoea on exertion.
- Fatigue.
- Orthopnoea and paroxysmal dyspnoea occur as disease progresses.
- Right heart failure may complicate left heart failure.

### SIGNS

- A wide pulse pressure occurs (difference between systolic and diastolic) and manifests in a number of ways:
  - Collapsing (water-hammer) pulse
  - Corrigan's sign – visible carotid pulsations in the neck

- De Musset's sign – nodding of the head in time with the heart beat
- Duroziez's sign – 'to and fro' murmur in the femoral artery on distal occlusion
- Quincke's sign – nail bed pulsation
- Traube's sign – 'pistol shot' sounds over the femoral arteries
- Muller's sign – pulsation of the uvula
- The apex beat is laterally displaced and hyperdynamic.

---

**The murmur**

**Early diastolic murmur over the lower left sternal edge** is heard. It is accentuated when the patient leans forward and breathes out. S1 is soft and S2 may be loud (aortic root dilatation) or soft (valve abnormalities). An **Austin Flint murmur** may be present: a mid-diastolic murmur due to a regurgitant jet vibrating the anterior mitral valve leaflet and causing turbulence of flow entering the LV through the mitral valve from the LA.

---

INVESTIGATIONS

| ECG | LVH with strain |
|---|---|
| CXR | Cardiomegaly and dilatation of the ascending aorta |
| Echocardiography | LV dilatation may be apparent (see Figure 8.3) Severity can be assessed: <br> • Valve abnormality <br> • Width of the regurgitant jet <br> • Reversal of diastolic flow in the descending aorta |

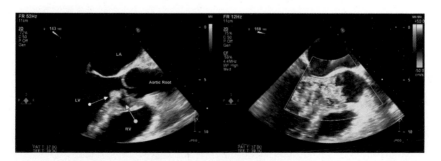

**Figure 8.3** Aortic regurgitation. Mid-oesophageal view of aortic valve on trans-oesophageal echocardiogram. In this three-chamber view, the right coronary cusp (RCC) has a significant vegetation burden (white arrow) and this has tethered the cusp severely resulting in flail RCC. This is resulting in severe aortic regurgitation directed towards the anterior mitral valve leaflet. There is also a fistula in the right coronary sinus (yellow arrow) with colour Doppler flow in it.

Cardiology and the cardiovascular system

### TREATMENT

- Patients may require medical therapy:
    - ACE inhibitors or ARBs may be beneficial in hypertensive patients with AR and heart failure.
    - Beta-blockers slow aortic root dilatation in patients with Marfan's syndrome.
- Indications for surgical treatment:
    - NYHA class III or IV heart failure (see Section 5.2)
    - Patients with NYHA class II failure with preserved function but with either:
        - Progressive LV dilatation
        - Declining ejection fraction
        - Declining exercise tolerance
    - Patients with LV ejection fractions less than 50%

## COMBINED AORTIC VALVE DISEASE

- Often both stenosis and regurgitation coexist.
- Echocardiography allows the contribution of each lesion to the flow to be assessed but concomitant regurgitation increases trans-aortic velocity and may over-estimate the severity of the stenosis as judged by Doppler.

# 8.5 MITRAL VALVE

## MITRAL VALVE STENOSIS

### CAUSES

- The most common cause for mitral stenosis is rheumatic heart disease.
- Age-related calcification can also occur.

### SYMPTOMS

- Often asymptomatic in the early stages.
- The predominant symptom is shortness of breath.
- Haemoptysis is reported by some patients, most likely due to raised pulmonary pressures.
- Palpitations due to atrial fibrillation are common.

---

## MICRO-facts

**Pulmonary hypertension** is defined as a mean pulmonary arterial pressure greater than 25 mmHg that may occur due to various causes and results in progressive right heart failure through increased pulmonary vascular resistance. Mitral stenosis is classified as a group II cause of pulmonary hypertension in the WHO classification.

---

*Cardiology and the cardiovascular system*

## SIGNS

- Signs of pulmonary congestion appear before eventual RV failure.
- Right heart failure may cause RV heave and elevated JVP.
- Malar flush is a dusky appearance over the cheeks associated with high pressures in the pulmonary vasculature.
- An irregular pulse due to atrial fibrillation.
- Apex beat is not usually displaced but may be tapping in nature.

---

**The murmur**
A 'rumbling' mid-diastolic murmur is heard at the apex. It increases at the end of diastole, accentuated in the left lateral position if the patient is in sinus rhythm. S1 is loud with an opening snap; S2 can increase in volume as pulmonary hypertension develops. The longer the murmur duration, the more severe the disease.

---

## INVESTIGATIONS

| ECG | AF common |
| --- | --- |
| | If sinus rhythm, P mitrale from LA dilatation (see Chapter 12, P wave section) Signs of RV hypertrophy |
| **CXR** | Calcification of the valve leaflets may be visible Look for signs of pulmonary congestion |
| **Echocardiography** | A swirling appearance of blood in the LA is reported Colour flow and Doppler modes allow quantification of flow through the valve and the pressure gradient between the LA and LV |

- Severity is assessed by valve areas and gradient as per EAE/ASE recommendations

| | MILD | MODERATE | SEVERE |
| --- | --- | --- | --- |
| Mitral valve area (cm$^2$) | >1.5 | 1.0–1.5 | <1.0 |
| Median pressure gradient (mmHg) | <5 | 5–10 | >10 |

Cardiology and the cardiovascular system

**MICRO-references**
Baumgartner H, Hung J, Bermejo J, et al. Echocardiographic assessment of valve stenosis: EAE/ASE recommendations for clinical practice. *European Journal of Echocardiography* 2009; 10(1): 1–25. ESC/EACTS Guidelines. Guidelines on the management of valvular heart disease. *European Heart Journal* 2012; 33: 2451–2496.

## MANAGEMENT

- AF should be managed according to standard protocols.
- Diuretics and long-acting nitrates can be given for symptomatic relief of breathlessness.
- Beta-blockers and rate-limiting calcium channel blockers lengthen diastole and therefore increase exercise tolerance.
- Balloon valvotomy may be attempted to enlarge the valve area:
  - A balloon is inserted into the valve orifice and inflated.
  - This may be suitable in valves with pliable cusps with little calcification.
  - Should not be used if there is any associated mitral regurgitation.
- Surgery aims to either repair or replace the valve:
  - Surgery is indicated for patients who are significantly symptomatic or:
    - Suffer episodes of acute pulmonary oedema
    - Recurrent emboli
    - Pulmonary oedema in pregnancy
    - Deterioration due to AF even with maximal medical therapy
- Even in the absence of AF, it may be necessary to consider anti-coagulation as there is a risk of atrial thrombosis and embolization.

## MITRAL VALVE REGURGITATION

### Chronic mitral regurgitation

#### CAUSES

- Chronic mitral regurgitation may be due to:
  - Degenerative disease in the elderly
  - Rheumatic heart disease
  - Infective endocarditis
  - LV dilatation stretching the mitral annulus

#### SYMPTOMS

- Classically presents with slowly progressive fatigue and dyspnoea on exertion

#### SIGNS

- Pulse is of normal volume (often high volume).
  - AF is common.

- JVP is normal unless right-sided failure occurs.
- The apex beat is prominent, sustained and displaced downwards and laterally.

---

**The murmur**

A **pansystolic** murmur is heard at the apex, radiating to the axilla and left subscapular region. S1 is quiet and S2 may be split. The Valsalva manoeuvre can accentuate the murmur. The presence of a third heart sound (due to rapid ventricular filling), and the duration and intensity of the sound are signs of severity.

A late systolic murmur and mid-systolic click are characteristic of valve prolapse.

---

INVESTIGATIONS

| ECG | AF common<br>In sinus rhythm, P mitrale from LA dilatation<br>(see Chapter 12, P wave section) |
|---|---|
| CXR | Enlargement of LA<br>Calcified valve from rheumatic heart disease |
| Echocardiography | Can show thickening of the valve leaflets<br>Prolapsing leaflets may also be visible<br>Colour flow Doppler useful for showing regurgitant jet |

MANAGEMENT

- Medical therapy focuses on treating any associated heart failure.
- In contrast to other valves of the heart, the mitral valve may often be repaired in preference to replacement.
- Surgery is indicated:
  - In severe regurgitation if symptomatic despite medical therapy
  - In severe regurgitation with deteriorating LV function or dilatation even if asymptomatic, i.e.:
    - Reduction of ejection fraction <60% or
    - LV end systolic dimension >45 mm

Mitral valve prolapse

- Prolapse of one or both valve leaflets into the LA during systole is the most common valve abnormality.
- Normally associated with trivial mitral regurgitation and can lead to the same complications as mitral regurgitation.
- Usually requires only reassurance but some patients who develop significant regurgitation may require valve repair.

Cardiology and the cardiovascular system

> **The murmur**
> A mid-systolic click and high-pitched late systolic murmur is heard loudest at the apex.

## ACUTE MITRAL VALVE REGURGITATION

In acute mitral regurgitation, the changes in haemodynamics are not tolerated as compensatory ventricular and atrial changes have not occurred.

### CAUSES

- Most often due to papillary muscle rupture following myocardial infarction
- Infective endocarditis
- Myxomatous degeneration causing chordae rupture

### SYMPTOMS

- Acute pulmonary oedema with dyspnoea
- Shock

### SIGNS

- The systolic murmur is often short and soft.
- A fourth heart sound may be heard.

### INVESTIGATIONS

| ECG | Check for ST segment changes indicating acute MI |
|---|---|
| CXR | Pulmonary oedema<br>Normal sized heart |
| Echocardiography | Flail leaflets may be apparent if regurgitation is due to papillary muscle or chordal rupture |

### MANAGEMENT

- Often emergency surgery is warranted following medical therapy, and intra-aortic balloon pumping may be used for haemodynamic stabilization.

## MICRO-facts

Intra-aortic balloon pump should be avoided in aortic regurgitation as it worsens the pressure gradient between the aorta and LV.

# 8.6 TRICUSPID VALVE

## TRICUSPID VALVE STENOSIS

- Tricuspid stenosis is rare and nearly always due to rheumatic heart disease.
- It is associated with carcinoid syndrome.
- Mitral stenosis often coexists leading to mid-diastolic and pre-systolic murmurs.
- Rheumatic lesions appear similar to those that occur on the mitral valve:
  - Thickened valve cusps
  - Chordae shortened and thickened
- The narrowed valve obstructs flow from the RA to the RV.
- This leads to RA and vena cava dilatation:
  - P pulmonale on ECG (in sinus rhythm)
  - JVP displays large 'a' waves
  - Hepatic engorgement and ascites
  - Peripheral oedema

## TRICUSPID VALVE REGURGITATION

- Functional tricuspid regurgitation is a common consequence of right-sided failure and pulmonary hypertension caused by stretching of the tricuspid annulus.
- Features are due to a large volume of blood passing back into the atrium.
  - Leads to:
    - Pulsatile, engorged liver
    - Ascites
    - JVP with giant 'v' waves and a prominent 'y' descent
    - Parasternal heave and loud P2
    - Pansystolic murmur at the lower left sternal edge (increased by inspiration)
- Repair or replacement of the valve may also be necessary.

# 8.7 PULMONARY VALVE

- Pulmonary valve disease is relatively uncommon.
- Congenital pulmonary stenosis is the most common cause.
- Pulmonary stenosis may also be due to:
  - Rheumatic heart disease
  - Malignant carcinoid
- Pulmonary regurgitation occurs due to pulmonary hypertension and annular dilatation.
- **Graham Steel murmur** is an early diastolic murmur heard in the pulmonary area.
- Valve replacement is rarely required but may be indicated in intractable right-sided failure.

# 8.8 VALVE REPLACEMENT

- Full pre- and post-operative assessment, baseline investigations and lifelong follow-up with a cardiologist are required.
- The choice of which type of valve to implant is based on many factors.

## BIOPROSTHETIC

- Usually avoided in the under 40s as valvular degeneration can occur after 10–15 years.
- Valves undergo endothelialization so there is a low thrombotic risk after the first 3 months:
  - As such, anti-coagulation can usually be avoided in the long term.

## MECHANICAL VALVES

- These carry a low risk of valve degeneration and are therefore useful in any age.
- Can be effective for 20–30 years.
- Lifelong anti-coagulation is required.

---

**MICRO-print**

Valve degeneration develops 10–15 years after valve implantation, more commonly in bioprosthetic valves. It can involve:

- Weakness or tearing of the valve
- Scar formation and thickening of the valve leaflets
- Accelerated calcification
- Thrombosis

Deterioration is accelerated in bioprosthetic valves, particularly in:

- Younger patients (and particularly fast in children)
- Chronic renal failure
- Hyperparathyroidism

---

## COMPLICATIONS

- **Thromboembolism and anti-coagulation-related problems account for the majority of complications**
- Haemolytic anaemia
- Primary valve failure – acute or chronic
- Prosthetic valve endocarditis:
  - Defined as early (occurring within 60 days) or late
  - Caused by haematogenous spread of bacteria
  - In 'early' cases may be due to peri-operative contamination

## MICRO-facts

Features of prosthetic valve endocarditis include:

- Ring abscess in mechanical valves
- Scar rupture
- Perivalvular leak with sudden haemolytic anaemia
- Myocardial abscess
- Perforation of a bioprosthetic valve
- Systemic effects

### MICRO-case

A 70-year-old woman saw her GP after experiencing episodes of chest pain when walking to the shops. The episodes had gradually worsened in severity over 6 months. The chest pain was pressing in nature and was alleviated by rest. She also experienced some 'funny episodes' associated with the chest pain. During these episodes, she felt faint and had to sit down; once she had fainted after walking up a steep hill. She had also experienced palpitations and episodes of breathlessness over the last month. She had a long history of hypertension, which was currently stable on treatment with verapamil. She had no other medical history and had not had chest pain in the past. The chest pain and syncopal episodes were beginning to restrict her activities. On examination, she had a slow rising, irregularly irregular pulse of 79 bpm with a blood pressure of 110/90. There was an ejection systolic murmur over the second intercostal space at the right sternal edge. The murmur radiated to the carotids. The apex beat was heaving. The findings were suggestive of aortic stenosis with atrial fibrillation. The GP referred her to the cardiology clinic, where she had an ECG and echocardiogram. These tests demonstrated aortic stenosis with a reduced area across the aortic valve due to calcification (area 0.6 cm$^2$, gradient 70 mmHg). There was left ventricular hypertrophy, but left ventricular systolic function was good. Due to the functional impairment caused by her symptoms, she had an aortic valve replacement.

### Points to consider:

- Angina can have several causes other than coronary artery disease.
- Nitrates should not be prescribed in patients with severe aortic stenosis as they may substantially decrease the preload and this could lead to a profoundly reduced output in the presence of stenosis.
- Valve disease can cause both arrhythmias and heart failure.
- Cardiovascular examination is important in any patient with cardiac symptoms. Murmurs are an important indicator or cause of cardiac disease that can be easily detected.

Cardiology and the cardiovascular system

# 9 Congenital heart disease

## 9.1 EARLY CIRCULATION

### EMBRYOLOGY

- The heart develops from mesodermal cells.
- Defects in heart formation arise between 3 and 6 weeks gestation.
- The heart begins to beat at 22 days.
- In the foetal circulation, the placenta is the main source of oxygenation as only 10% of blood passes through the lung.
- Three left to right shunts allow the foetal circulation to bypass the lungs and liver (see Figure 9.1):
  - Ductus arteriosus
  - Ductus venosus
  - Foramen ovale

> ## MICRO-facts
>
> The ductus arteriosus is kept open in utero by low partial oxygen levels and high levels of circulating prostaglandins (maternal non-steroidal anti-inflammatory drug use can induce foetal closure).
>
> **Duct-dependent defects:** some congenital defects rely on the ductus arteriosus for pulmonary or systemic circulation when the normal sequence of blood flow through the heart is interrupted. These include:
>
> | SYSTEMIC CIRCULATION | PULMONARY CIRCULATION |
> | --- | --- |
> | Hypoplastic left heart | Critical pulmonary stenosis Pulmonary atresia |
> | Critical aortic stenosis | Tricuspid atresia |
> | Coarctation of the aorta | Tetralogy of Fallot |
> | Interruption of the aorta | Transposition of the great arteries |
>
> *continued...*

> *continued...*
>
> These lesions can present suddenly when the ductus arteriosus closes in the first few days of life, resulting in cardiogenic shock. The duct can be kept patent by **prostaglandin E2** (side effects include hypotension and apnoeas).

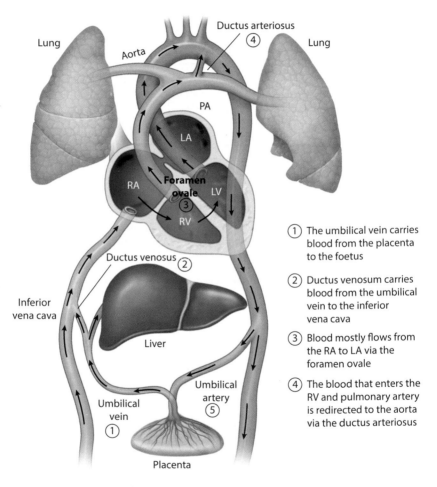

① The umbilical vein carries blood from the placenta to the foetus

② Ductus venosum carries blood from the umbilical vein to the inferior vena cava

③ Blood mostly flows from the RA to LA via the foramen ovale

④ The blood that enters the RV and pulmonary artery is redirected to the aorta via the ductus arteriosus

**Figure 9.1** Neonatal circulation.

## CHANGES AT BIRTH

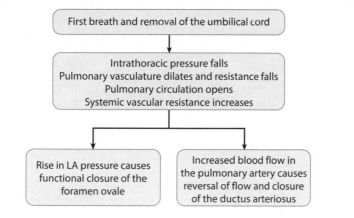

# 9.2 PATHOLOGY

Congenital disease can be divided into four groups:
1. Communications:
   a. Abnormal shunting of blood between the pulmonary and systemic circulations causing progressive damage.
2. Cyanotic:
   a. Causes cyanosis through a variety of mechanisms
   b. Usually a right to left shunt
3. Obstructive:
   a. Obstructing the smooth flow of blood and creating back pressure
4. Complex:
   a. When anomalies in these categories are grouped together as an entity

# 9.3 COMMUNICATIONS

## ATRIAL SEPTAL DEFECTS (ASD)

- ASDs are relatively common and occur frequently in isolation.

### Patent foramen ovale (PFO)

- Remnant of the normal foetal circulation that may persist in up to 25% of people.
- Linked to unexplained thrombotic events in the young as it may allow passage of a venous thrombus into the arterial circulation (known as paradoxical embolism), e.g. deep vein thrombosis causing a stroke.

### Secundum atrial septal defects

- Defect of the fossa ovalis that does not affect the atrioventricular valves (see Figure 9.2).
- It is the most common form of ASD.

Cardiology and the cardiovascular system

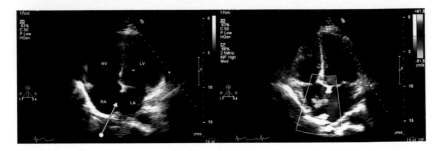

**Figure 9.2** Atrial septal defect. Apical four-chamber view on transthoracic echo-cardiogram with colour Doppler to confirm a large secundum ASD (white arrow) with left to right shunt.

## Primum atrial septal defects

- A defect occurring lower down in the atrial septum
- Involves the atrioventricular junction and is associated with valve incompetence

## Sinus venosus atrial septal defects

- A rare defect occurring in the upper part of the atrial septum
- Usually adjacent to the superior vena cava
- Normally associated with anomalous pulmonary venous drainage

### SYMPTOMS

- PFO may cause no symptoms.
- Secundum defects are often asymptomatic before the age of 30 years.
- When symptomatic can cause breathlessness and fatigue.
- Palpitations in the presence of atrial fibrillation.

### SIGNS

- Small arterial pulse.
- Wide, fixed split of the second heart sound.
- A systolic murmur due to high pulmonary flow may occur.
- Primum defects cause left-sided atrioventricular valve regurgitation.
- Atrial fibrillation is common in older patients with ASD.

### INVESTIGATIONS

| ECG | Partial or complete right bundle branch block<br>Right axis deviation in secundum defect<br>Left axis deviation in primum defects |
|-----|-----------------------------------------------------------------------------------------------------------------------------------|
| CXR | Cardiomegaly and pulmonary plethora |

*Continued*

| Echocardiography | Right-sided chambers are dilated |
|---|---|
| | Significant secundum defects may show a paradoxical septal movement due to volume overloaded RV |
| | The abnormal valve is visible in primum defects |
| | Blood flow across the inter-atrial septum may be seen on Doppler or with bubble contrast |
| | Trans-oesophageal echo may be necessary to demonstrate a PFO |

## MANAGEMENT

- Closure of all significant secundum defects with RV volume overload is recommended:
  - Percutaneous closure is an option in secundum defects.
- Primum defects require surgical closure often with mitral/tricuspid valve repair:
  - Indicated if symptomatic or a large shunt is present.
- Closure of PFO is controversial unless thrombotic events have occurred.
- Closure before age 20 years almost abolishes the risk of late complications like AF.

## VENTRICULAR SEPTAL DEFECTS (VSDS)

- VSDs are the second most common congenital cardiac lesion after bicuspid aortic valves (see Figure 9.3).
- May occur in isolation or in combination with other abnormalities.

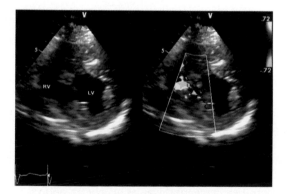

**Figure 9.3** Ventricular septal defect. Post-myocardial infarction VSD is apparent in mid-septum secondary to wall rupture. There is a large left to right shunt across it, evident on colour Doppler.

- There are four components to the ventricular septum:
  - Trabecular septum (extends to the apex)
  - Inlet septum (between the atrioventricular valves)
  - Outlet septum (immediately below the great arteries)
  - Membranous septum (below the aortic root)
- Defects may occur in any of these regions but the membranous septum is the most common location.

### Symptoms

- Effects depend on the size of the defect; large defects cause heart failure early in life.

### Signs

- Evidence of heart failure and failure to thrive in large left to right shunts.
- Large-volume pulse.
- Loud pansystolic murmur at the lower left sternal edge.
- Mid-diastolic murmur due to high flow through the mitral valve.
- Eventually leads to pulmonary hypertension (right ventricular heave; loud P2).
- Small defects cause loud murmurs but no signs of heart failure (Maladie de Roger).

### Investigations

| ECG | May be normal in small defects Deep narrow Q waves and tall R waves in V1–V3 (RVH) Partial or complete RBBB |
| --- | --- |
| CXR | Cardiomegaly and pulmonary plethora |
| Echocardiography | Right-sided volume loading (dilated RV and RA) Allows visualization of exact anatomical position |

### Management

- Therapy depends on the expected prognosis.
- Failure to thrive or heart failure in infancy should prompt closure of the defect.
- Infants with good weight gain may be observed and treatment may be delayed.
- In large defects, surgery is the treatment of choice:
  - Early surgery may prevent pulmonary hypertension.
  - However, if pulmonary hypertension has occurred surgery may worsen it.
- In small defects, percutaneous therapies may be an option.
- Many patients with small defects have a normal life expectancy but an increased risk of infective endocarditis.

## MICRO-facts

Eisenmenger syndrome describes the sequence of events that occur in patients with left to right shunts. Increased pulmonary blood flow leads to vasoconstriction of the pulmonary vascular bed. Right heart pressures increase and pulmonary flow decreases. High RV pressure causes reversal of the shunt and cyanosis and symptoms of hypoxaemia occur. Pulmonary vasodilators may be an option but often a heart and lung transplant is required.

## MICRO-facts

Endocardial cushion defect (complete AVSD) is the combination of an ASD, VSD and valve abnormalities. It has a strong association with Down's syndrome and necessitates surgical correction as soon as possible.

## PERSISTENT DUCTUS ARTERIOSUS (PDA)

- In the foetal circulation, the *ductus arteriosus* permits blood to flow from the pulmonary artery to the aorta:
  - Usually closes within days of birth
  - Often remains open in premature neonates and leads to blood flow from the aorta directly to the pulmonary circulation

### SYMPTOMS

- May cause heart failure in the first weeks of life.
- Commonly partial closure occurs and the PDA may then be found on routine examination or become problematic when:
  - It becomes a focus for infective *endoarteritis*.
  - The increased pulmonary blood flow from the aorta leads to failure.
  - It may lead to pulmonary hypertension.

### SIGNS

- If a large PDA is present, a collapsing pulse may result.
- Low diastolic blood pressure.
- Continuous 'mechanical' murmur loudest in the second intercostal space on the left.

Cardiology and the cardiovascular system

### INVESTIGATIONS

| ECG | LVH |
|---|---|
| CXR | Cardiomegaly and aortic/pulmonary artery dilatation |
| Echocardiography | The pulmonary artery is dilated<br>The duct may not be visible on echocardiography<br>The shunt is identified by Doppler showing<br>  abnormal flow |

### MANAGEMENT

- Often PDAs may be closed percutaneously.
- In premature infants with symptomatic PDA, indomethacin may aid medical closure.
- Surgery is reserved for very large defects causing heart failure.

## 9.4 CYANOTIC

### TETRALOGY OF FALLOT

- Tetralogy of Fallot is the most common abnormality in cyanotic heart disease (see Figure 9.4).

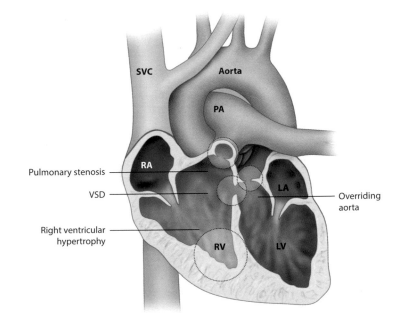

**Figure 9.4** Tetralogy of Fallot.

- It describes a syndrome with four cardiac manifestations:
  - Infundibular muscular pulmonary stenosis
  - VSD
  - Overriding aorta
  - RV hypertrophy

## SYMPTOMS

- Symptoms depend on the degree of pulmonary stenosis:
  - If severe there is little pulmonary blood flow and a large right to left shunt occurs.
- May present similar to a large VSD (left to right shunt):
  - Eventually, there may be a reversal of the shunt leading to central desaturation.
- Hypercyanotic spells are caused by muscular spasm around the area of obstruction, which may lead to myocardial infarction or cerebrovascular accidents:
  - These episodes may be alleviated by squatting.

## SIGNS

- Often there may be features of external dysmorphia.
- Central cyanosis and clubbing are classic features.
- Low volume arterial pulses may be present.
- Loud systolic murmur with thrill in second and third intercostal spaces.
- Single second heart sound due to the pulmonary component being inaudible.

## INVESTIGATIONS

| ECG | RV hypertrophy (partial or complete RBBB, dominant R waves V1–V3) |
|-----|------------------------------------------------------------------|
| CXR | Boot-shaped heart presenting as a concavity on the left border where the pulmonary artery normally arises<br>Decreased pulmonary vasculature |
| Echocardiogram | May show the abnormalities |
| Angiography | May show distal pulmonary artery abnormalities poorly seen on echo<br>Abnormal coronary anatomy may coexist |

## MANAGEMENT

- Can be fatal without surgical intervention.
- Type of surgery depends on the severity and exact anatomy of the disease.
- Correction is by closure of the VSD and relief of right ventricular outflow tract obstruction (pulmonary regurgitation is common postoperatively).

Cardiology and the cardiovascular system

## TRANSPOSITION OF THE GREAT ARTERIES

- Transposition of the great arteries is the most common cardiac cause of cyanosis immediately after birth.
- Quick diagnosis is essential as the condition can prove rapidly fatal.
- Reversal of the origins of the great vessels (see Figure 9.5):
  - Aorta arises from the RV.
  - Pulmonary artery arises from the LV.
- There are, therefore, separate systemic and pulmonary circulations.
- Incompatible with life unless coexists with one of:
  - Patent foramen ovale
  - Atrial septal defect
  - Ventricular septal defect
  - Persistent ductus arteriosus

### Signs

- Cyanosis usually develops at birth or shortly after.

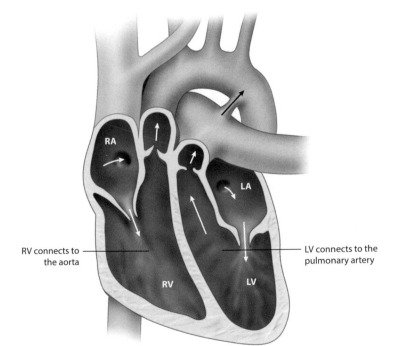

**Figure 9.5** Greater artery transposition.

Cardiology and the cardiovascular system

INVESTIGATIONS

| CXR | Usually normal at birth but rapidly changes to show cardiomegaly and increased lung vascularity |
|---|---|
| **Echocardiogram** | Delineates the abnormalities |

TREATMENT

- Balloon septostomy after echocardiographical diagnosis:
  - A tear is produced in the atrial septum.
  - Allows mixing of blood from the two circulations and so does not cure cyanosis.
- Ultimate management is surgical:
  - Previously atrial switch operations (Senning or Mustard procedures).
  - Current arterial switch procedures allow anatomical and physiological correction of flow.

# 9.5 OBSTRUCTIVE

## COARCTATION OF THE AORTA

- Coarctation normally occurs in the distal aortic arch.
- The most common site is immediately distal to the origin of the left subclavian artery and proximal to the PDA.
- Two presentations occur:
  - Critical neonatal coarctation:
    - Often presents with cardiovascular collapse after the PDA closes.
    - Intravenous prostaglandin reopens the duct allowing time to implement more permanent management.
  - Later presentations in infancy or adulthood.

SYMPTOMS

- Frequently asymptomatic if does not present with critical coarctation

SIGNS

- Lower blood pressure in the lower body and hypertension in the upper limbs.
- Radial-femoral delay.
- Flow murmur may be heard over the coarctation often in the back around the left scapula.
- Collateralization occurs and vessels may be visible.

INVESTIGATIONS

| ECG | May show LVH in adulthood |
|---|---|
| CXR | Normal in early childhood<br>Characteristic changes are:<br>• Abnormal aortic knuckle<br>• Enlarged left subclavian artery<br>• Post-coarctation dilation<br>Notching of the ribs due to enlarged intercostal arteries |
| Echocardiography | 50–85% of patients with coarctation have a bicuspid aortic valve<br>TOE may demonstrate the abnormality |
| CT or MRI | Best evaluation |

TREATMENT OPTIONS

- Surgery: resection of coarctation and interpositional graft (should be performed early as long-term results worsen with age at surgery)
- Balloon angioplasty: poor outcomes and largely replaced by stenting and surgery
- Stenting: less effective than surgery but may have a role in patients with recurrent coarctation post-surgery

## PULMONARY STENOSIS

- Pulmonary stenosis is almost always of a congenital nature.
- Occurs as an isolated defect or a complex malformation.
- Obstruction can occur at a number of levels of the RV outflow tract and multilevel obstruction may occur:
  - Valvular obstruction (most common)
  - Subvalvular obstruction
  - Supravalvular obstruction (least common)

### MICRO-facts
Pulmonary stenosis may exist with many childhood syndromes – most commonly Noonan syndrome.

SYMPTOMS

- May lead to RV failure.
- Right to left shunts and cyanosis may occur if there is a coexisting PFO or ASD.

Cardiology and the cardiovascular system

### SIGNS

- Pulse is usually normal.
- JVP may show large 'a' waves if severe.
- Thrill in the second left intercostal space.
- Left parasternal heave if ventricular hypertrophy has occurred.
- May hear ejection 'click' and a mid-systolic ejection murmur.
- Wide splitting of the second heart sound as the disease progresses.

### INVESTIGATIONS

| ECG | RV hypertrophy |
|---|---|
| CXR | Dilatation of the pulmonary artery distal to the stenosis |
| Echocardiography | Gold standard for diagnosis and allows planning for any intervention |

### TREATMENT

- Mild disease may be observed.
- Treatment may prevent progression of RV hypertrophy.
- Balloon valvuloplasty may enlarge the valve orifice.
- Surgery may be used to enlarge or replace the valve.

## 9.6 COMPLEX

- Single ventricle circulations are rare.
- The circulation exists as a single physiological chamber.
- The most common abnormality is tricuspid atresia.

### TRICUSPID ATRESIA

- Absence of the normal atrioventricular connection on the right side of the heart (see Figure 9.6).
- Right ventricle is usually small.
- Only compatible with life if it coexists with an ASD.
- Often exists with other congenital pathology.
- Long-term management is with an operation to create a Fontan circulation:
  - Vena cava is connected to the pulmonary arteries.
  - Pulmonary circulation relies on venous circulation.

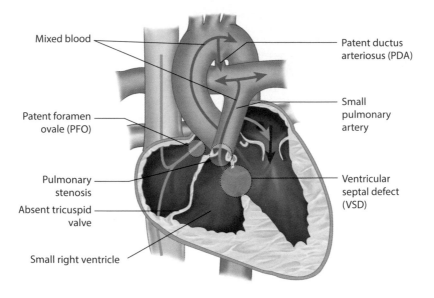

**Figure 9.6** Tricuspid atresia.

## GENETIC ABNORMALITIES AND ASSOCIATED CONGENITAL SYNDROMES

| DISORDER | INHERITANCE | CHARACTERISTIC CARDIAC FEATURE |
|---|---|---|
| Down's syndrome | Sporadic: trisomy 21 | AVSD |
| William's syndrome | Sporadic: microdeletion | Supravalvular aortic stenosis |
| DiGeorge syndrome | Sporadic: microdeletion | Interruption of the aortic arch and tetralogy of Fallot |
| Noonan syndrome | Autosomal dominant | Pulmonary stenosis and ASD |
| Marfan's syndrome | Autosomal dominant | Floppy mitral valve, aortic root dilatation with AR, dissection or aneurysm |
| Turner syndrome | Sporadic: XO and XXO | Coarctation of the aorta and VSD |
| Ciliary dyskinesia | Autosomal recessive | Association with dextrocardia and situs inversus |

Cardiology and the cardiovascular system

## TERATOGENS ASSOCIATED WITH CONGENITAL CARDIAC DISEASE

| DRUGS | INFECTION | MATERNAL MORBIDITY |
|---|---|---|
| Lithium – Ebstein's anomaly | Rubella – PDA | Diabetes mellitus |
| Anti-epileptic drugs | Toxoplasmosis | Systemic lupus erythematosus – congenital heart block |
| Alcohol or illicit drug exposure | Cytomegalovirus | |

### MICRO-case

A 9-month-old boy was taken to the GP by his parents who were worried about his breathing. He had been suffering from cold symptoms for 2 days and then his breathing appeared to have deteriorated over the preceding 24 hours. On examination, he was extremely breathless with a respiratory rate of 50 breaths per minute, and he was using accessory muscles. On auscultation wheezes were heard bilaterally. He was immediately admitted to the local hospital, where he was diagnosed with, and treated for, severe bronchiolitis. While recovering in hospital a new pansystolic murmur was heard at the lower left sternal edge. Review of the history revealed an uneventful gestational period and birth with no defects detected on pre-natal screening or routine childhood surveillance. However, since birth he had dropped one centile on his growth chart. On direct questioning, his parents stated that he appeared breathless prior to this episode, particularly while eating, but otherwise seemed to be a well child. A chest radiograph showed prominent pulmonary vessels and an echocardiogram demonstrated a large VSD. ECG was normal. He was referred for closure of the defect but while waiting for surgery fell another centile on his growth chart.

**Points to consider:**

- Congenital heart disease may be diagnosed at several stages including in the prenatal or neonatal period or in childhood or adulthood.
- Common presentations of communicating congenital heart defects include breathlessness and failure to thrive.
- Children with heart defects should be examined for other abnormalities that may form part of a syndrome or sequence.

Cardiology and the cardiovascular system

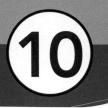

# Hypertension

## 10.1 MEASURING BLOOD PRESSURE

- Avoid stimulants such as caffeine, hot baths or exercise prior to measurement.
- BP should be taken sitting (may be taken lying and standing to measure a postural drop).
- Inflate the cuff to 20 mmHg above the point at which the radial pulse is not palpable.
- Gradually deflate the cuff while auscultating over the brachial artery.
- When the first regular pulsation is heard, this is the systolic BP (first Korotkoff sound).
- When the sounds disappear, this is the diastolic BP (fifth Korotkoff sound).

## AMBULATORY BLOOD PRESSURE MONITORING

Patients with an isolated BP of >140/90 mmHg should be offered ABPM.

- ABPM records readings in waking hours as the patient continues their normal routine.
- An average of at least 14 readings is taken.
- Accurate for confirming hypertension and preventing unnecessary treatment.
- Home BP monitoring should be offered to patients who cannot tolerate ABPM.

# 10.2 CLASSIFICATION OF HYPERTENSION

- **Stage 1 hypertension:** clinic BP is 140/90 mmHg or higher, ABPM 135/85 mmHg average or higher.
- **Stage 2 hypertension:** clinic BP is 160/100 mmHg or higher, ABPM 150/95 mmHg average or higher.
- **Severe hypertension:** clinic systolic BP is 180 mmHg or higher, or clinic diastolic BP is 110 mmHg or higher.

## PRIMARY HYPERTENSION

- 'Idiopathic' hypertension
- Responsible for more than 95% of hypertension

### MECHANISMS

A number of factors have been shown to influence the risk of developing hypertension:

- *Genetic*
  - Evidence appears to support the role of a number of genes.
- *Dietary*
  - Association with increased weight.
  - A low salt diet may protect against the development of hypertension.
  - Weight loss in obese patients reduces BP.
  - Association with regular and excess alcohol intake.
- *Physical activity*
  - Regular physical activity reduces BP.
- *Hormonal*
  - Theorized that defects in the adrenergic and renin–angiotensin systems may play a role.
- *Haemodynamic*
  - Baroreceptor function is altered in hypertensive patients.
  - No bradycardic response to rising BP.

## SECONDARY HYPERTENSION

- Secondary hypertension is responsible for less than 5% of cases.

### MECHANISMS

- *Renal parenchymal disease*
    - Conditions that damage the kidney will cause hypertension.
    - Renal damage is often accelerated as a result.
    - Hypertension per se causes renal damage.
- *Renal vascular disease*
    - Renal artery stenosis is a recognized cause of hypertension:
        - Disease can be unilateral or bilateral.
        - In older patients, the cause is often atherosclerosis.
        - In younger patients, it may be due to fibromuscular dysplasia.
        - Decreased renal blood flow leads to increased production of renin and a rise in BP.
- *Pregnancy*
    - Hypertension can occur during pregnancy.
    - Most frequently in younger mothers.
    - Hypertension normalizes after delivery of the foetus.
    - Pregnancy may also worsen pre-existing hypertension.
    - Careful monitoring is necessary as hypertension may lead to pre-eclampsia.
    - A history of hypertension in pregnancy is associated with persistent hypertension in later life.
- *Coarctation of the aorta* (see Section 9.2)
    - A congenital defect narrowing the aorta distal to the left subclavian artery
    - Leads to raised pressures in the arms and low pressures in the legs
    - Activates the renin–aldosterone system
- *Drug induced*
    - Most commonly caused by the oral contraceptive pill
    - Corticosteroids
    - Erythropoietin
    - Ciclosporin
- *Endocrine*
    - **Primary aldosteronism** (Conn's syndrome):
        - High aldosterone and low renin levels.
        - Leads to sodium and water overload.
        - This normally results from an adrenal cortex adenoma.
        - Blood results show hypokalaemia and mild hypernatraemia.

- **Cushing's syndrome/disease:**
  - Results from excess cortisol.
  - Due to adrenal hyperplasia, adrenal tumours or excess administration of glucocorticoids.
  - Adrenal hyperplasia is most often due to ACTH production from a pituitary microadenoma (Cushing's syndrome).
- **Phaeochromocytoma:**
  - A tumour of the chromaffin tissue.
  - 90% arise in the adrenal glands, 10% elsewhere.
  - 10% are malignant and 10% are bilateral.
  - May present as a fluctuating BP, chest pain, tachycardia and sweating.

---

**MICRO-print**
Causes of secondary hypertension can be remembered as **REPAIR**:

| **R**enovascular | Renal artery stenosis |
|---|---|
| **E**ndocrine | Conn's syndrome, **C**ushing's syndrome, a**C**romegaly, phae**C**hromocytoma |
| **P**regnancy | |
| **A**ortic coarctation | |
| **I**atrogenic – drugs | Oral contraceptive pill, steroids, erythropoietin, ciclosporin |
| **R**enal parenchymal | |

---

## ACCELERATED HYPERTENSION

- Can be termed malignant hypertension.
- Typified by diastolic pressures of over 130 mmHg.
- Most commonly affects patients with secondary hypertension.
- Retinal haemorrhages and papilloedema are common.
- Cerebral oedema may occur, leading to hypertensive encephalopathy.
- Heart and renal failure may also occur.
- Urgent referral is necessary and intravenous therapies may be necessary to bring the BP under control (but not too quickly because of cerebral autoregulation).

INVESTIGATIONS

| Laboratory tests | Urinalysis | Send to look for protein using the albumin:creatinine ratio and look for microscopic haematuria using a dipstick test |
|---|---|---|
| | U&E | Check sodium and potassium which may signify an endocrine cause<br>Monitor renal function |
| | Blood glucose | Raised in undiagnosed diabetic patients |
| | Lipid profile | To quantify cardiovascular risk |
| ECG | | Look for evidence of LVH (see Figure 10.1) |
| Other | Fundoscopy | Look for hypertensive retinopathy |

---

**MICRO-print**

Hypertensive retinopathy can be divided into stages based on fundoscopic images:

| Stage 1 | Arteriolar narrowing and tortuosity 'Silver wiring' |
|---|---|
| Stage 2 | Arterio-venous nipping |
| Stage 3 | Cotton wool exudates<br>Flame and blot haemorrhages |
| Stage 4 | Papilloedema |

---

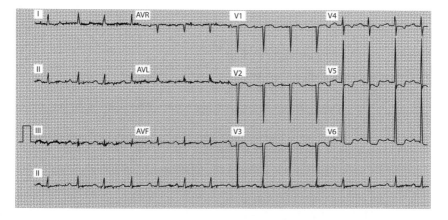

**Figure 10.1** ECG demonstrating LVH in precordial leads with repolarization defect.

Cardiology and the cardiovascular system

## COMPLICATIONS

Hypertension is usually asymptomatic; the damage caused is insidious and cumulative. A number of systems are affected by hypertension:

- Cardiac:
  - LVH arises due to increased stress on the ventricle and may lead to failure.
  - Coronary disease is more common in hypertensive patients.
  - Increased risk of sudden arrhythmic death.
- Renal:
  - Gradual development of renal impairment normally accompanies hypertension.
  - Microalbuminuria may lead to more severe proteinuria.
  - Renal replacement therapy may be needed as a result.
- Neurological:
  - Stroke and TIA are more common in hypertensive patients.
  - The retina is often affected and may show signs of hypertensive retinopathy.

## TREATMENT

- Offer anti-hypertensive drug treatment to people with stage 1 hypertension who have one or more of the following:
  - Target organ damage
  - Established cardiovascular disease
  - Renal disease
  - Diabetes mellitus
  - A 10-year cardiovascular risk equivalent to 20% or greater
- Offer anti-hypertensive drug treatment to people of any age with stage 2 hypertension.
- NICE 2011 guidelines should be used to guide treatment.

## CHOOSING ANTI-HYPERTENSIVE DRUG TREATMENT

### Step 1 Treatment (see Figure 10.2)

- For people aged under 55 years:
  - ACE inhibitor (ACEi) or
  - Low-cost angiotensin II receptor blockers (ARB) if an ACEi is not tolerated
- People aged over 55 years and for people of Afro-Caribbean origin of any age:
  - Calcium channel blocker (CCB) or
  - Thiazide-like diuretic if any of the following:
    - CCB is not suitable.
    - Evidence of heart failure.
    - High risk of heart failure.

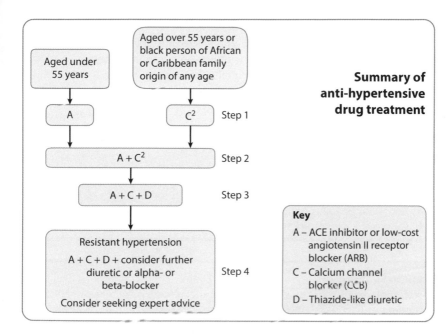

**Figure 10.2** NICE guidelines adapted flow chart.

- If treatment with a diuretic is being started, or changed, offer a thiazide-like diuretic, such as indapamide.

## Step 2 Treatment

- Two medications usually:
    - CCB in combination with ACEi or an ARB
    - Thiazide-like diuretic if any of the following:
        - CCB is not suitable.
        - Evidence of heart failure.
        - High risk of heart failure.
- For black people of African or Caribbean family origin:
    - ARB in preference to an ACEi used in combination with a CCB

## Step 3 Treatment

- Three medications:
    - ACEi or an ARB
    - CCB
    - Thiazide-like diuretic
- If BP 140/90 mmHg or higher after step 3 treatment:
    - If compliance with medication is assured then regard as resistant hypertension

## Step 4 Treatment of resistant hypertension

- Resistant hypertension requires referral to specialist management.
- Consider further diuretic therapy with low-dose spironolactone:
  - Only if the blood potassium level is 4.5 mmol/L or lower
- If the blood potassium level is higher than 4.5 mmol/L consider higher dose thiazide-like diuretic treatment.

### MICRO-facts

For people aged <40 years with stage 1 hypertension, consider specialist evaluation:

- Secondary causes of hypertension
- Detailed assessment of potential target organ damage

### MICRO-reference

National Institute for Health and Care Excellence. Hypertension. NICE guidelines [CG127]. London: National Institute for Health and Care Excellence, 2011.

### MICRO-case

A 60-year-old man attended his GP surgery for a 'well man' check. He attended infrequently and had not been seen by a doctor for 5 years. On examination with the practice nurse his BP was 154/96 mmHg and his urine dip was normal. He was a smoker (currently 10 per day, 35 pack-years) and overweight (BMI 29.5). He had no other past medical history. There was a positive family history of hypertension and his father had died of an MI at 67. On follow up with his GP, his cardiac examination and fundi were normal. He was advised about diet, exercise, smoking, alcohol and caffeine, and had ambulatory blood pressure monitoring (ABPM) arranged to assess his BP over 24 hours. Blood was taken for renal and liver function tests, fasting lipid profile and blood glucose level. He was seen again 2 weeks later. The ABPM took 16 measurements during normal waking hours and his average BP over that time was 152/95 mmHg. Using the results of the lipid profile, the average systolic BP, information taken from the history (smoking) and personal information (gender and age),

*continued...*

*continued...*

his 10-year cardiovascular risk was calculated showing a risk of 23% of death or MI in the next 10 years. He was advised strongly to stop smoking and referred to a nurse-led smoking cessation clinic. He was commenced on pharmacological therapy (atorvastatin and amlodipine) and arrangements were made for further BP monitoring to assess his response to treatment.

**Points to consider:**

- Several factors can cause an artificially elevated BP.
- Lifestyle advice is important as part of the treatment of high BP.
- Simple tests and examination can be used to exclude hypertension secondary to endocrine or renal causes.

Cardiology and the cardiovascular system

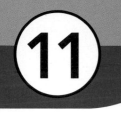

# 11 Diseases of the aorta

- The aorta is the largest artery of the body, connecting the heart to the arterial system.
- The wall of the aorta has three layers:
  - **Tunica intima** (endothelial lining)
  - **Tunica media** (elastic tissue)
  - **Tunica adventitia** (collagen with blood vessels and lymphatic drainage)

---

## MICRO-facts

The aorta has a high tensile strength due to the elastic fibres of the tunica media. This allows it to expand and contract in systole and diastole. This results in forward flow during diastole from elastic recoil.

---

- The aorta has both a thoracic and an abdominal component.
- The thoracic portion can be further divided:
  - **Ascending aorta** begins at the aortic root, supports the aortic valve and is the site of the sinuses of Valsalva from which the coronary arteries arise
  - **Aortic arch** is the origin of the brachiocephalic vessels providing blood to the arms and head
  - **Descending aorta** runs in the mediastinum and becomes the abdominal aorta at the diaphragm

## 11.1 ACUTE AORTIC DISSECTION

- This is an often fatal event in which a tear in the endothelium allows the tunica intima to be dissected away from the tunica media.
- This either occurs secondary to:
  - Spontaneous damage in a diseased aortic wall
  - Shearing forces placed on the aorta

- The most common causes of dissection in a diseased vessel:
  - Age-related weakness of collagen layers
  - Rupture of an atheromatous plaque
  - Common in inherited disorders of connective tissue, e.g. Marfan's syndrome, Ehlers–Danlos syndrome
  - Rare complication of pregnancy due to hormonal effects on the aorta

## SYMPTOMS

- Sudden, severe chest pain (tearing and either interscapular or anterior)
- May radiate to neck or arms
- Pain may be made worse on breathing and movement
- Nausea and vomiting
- Sweating
- Syncope

---

### MICRO-print
The signs and symptoms of acute aortic dissection can easily mimic those of a myocardial infarction. Moreover, in proximal dissections near the sinus of Valsalva, the dissection may involve the coronary ostia leading to myocardial ischaemia and myocardial infarction.

---

## SIGNS

- Hypertension (common finding due to previous history and response to the injury)
- Tachycardia
- Altered distal pulses (may be a difference in blood pressure between the arms – must be >20 mmHg in the elderly)
- Aortic regurgitation (may result if the dissection involves the aortic ring)
- Neurological manifestations including limb paraesthesiae/weakness – due to interruption of cerebral or spinal blood flow
- Pleural effusion (can result from bleeding into the pleural space)

---

### MICRO-facts
Some patients may be hypotensive at presentation, especially if the tear involves the aortic root, which can lead to bleeding into the pericardium and cardiac tamponade.

---

INVESTIGATIONS

| | | |
|---|---|---|
| **Laboratory tests** | FBC | Haemoglobin may drop if a significant amount of blood is lost but may be normal in acute loss |
| | U&E | Acute kidney injury may result from hypoperfusion of the kidneys |
| | D-Dimer | Elevation does not have 100% sensitivity, poor specificity |
| **CXR** | | May show widened mediastinum (unreliable) |
| **Echocardiogram** | | Damaged aortic root<br>Presence of a dissection flap<br>Unreliable imaging of the aortic arch and descending aorta on TTE |
| **CT** | | Useful to visualize the dissection flap<br>Will show intramural haematoma<br>Images the entirety of the aorta (see Figure 11.1) |
| **MRI** | | Similar sensitivity to CT<br>Longer scan times<br>Less readily available |
| **Angiography** | | Now usually superseded by CT scanning |

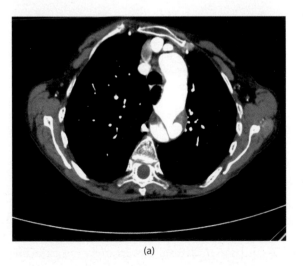

(a)

**Figure 11.1** CT imaging of an aortic dissection. Observe the double lumen forming as highlighted by contrast in these descending axial images of the (a) aortic arch. *(Continued)*

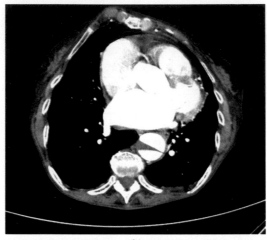

(b)

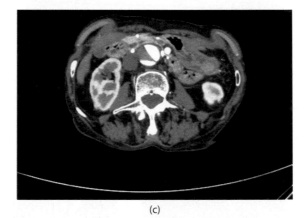

(c)

**Figure 11.1 (Continued)** CT imaging of an aortic dissection. Observe the double lumen forming as highlighted by contrast in these descending axial images of the (b) lower mediastinum and (c) abdomen.

### Classification

- Classification is by the Stanford system (see Figure 11.2):
  - **Type A** – proximal to the left subclavian artery (involves the ascending aorta)
  - **Type B** – distal to the left subclavian artery (no ascending aorta involvement)
- Type A dissections are thought to be more dangerous due to the possibility of coronary involvement and tamponade.

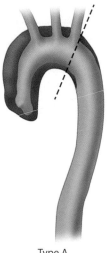 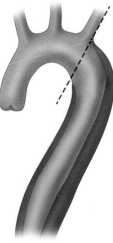

Type A                                      Type B

Figure 11.2 Diagram of the Stanford classification.

## MANAGEMENT

- **First-line treatment:**
  - Pain relief
  - Aggressive blood pressure control:
    - Avoid ACE inhibitors until renal arterial involvement is excluded as they may exacerbate renal failure.
- **Type A dissections** – surgery is the definitive management.
  - Repair or replacement of the aortic root and valve may also be necessary.
- **Type B dissections** – may be managed medically
  - Surgery does not decrease mortality but may be necessary if tissue ischaemia is present (e.g. involvement of renal or mesenteric vessels).
  - Covered stenting has become an option.
- Any surgery in dissection patients should be considered high risk with a high mortality and risk of complications.
- If dissection involves the pericardium, then death occurs rapidly from tamponade.

> **MICRO-print**
> Occasionally, thrombus within the wall of an artery may be found on imaging without any dissection flap. These intramural haematomata are managed medically and with follow-up imaging to look for resolution.

# 11.2 AORTIC ANEURYSMS

- An aneurysm is a dilatation of the wall in which all layers of the aorta are dilated.
- Normally occurs due to atherosclerosis and hypertension.
- Aneurysms gradually enlarge at a variable rate.
- Larger aneurysms are at a higher risk of rupture.
- Aneurysms most commonly affect the descending aorta.
- A false aneurysm does not involve all layers of the aorta, and the wall of the aneurysm is formed by a haematoma.

## SIGNS AND SYMPTOMS

- Often patients are asymptomatic with no clinical signs.
- May experience bouts of pain (the nature and site of pain depend on the location of the aneurysm).
- Hoarseness (may result due to stretching of the recurrent laryngeal nerve).
- Often hypertensive.
- Symptoms and signs of aortic regurgitation (may result from aortic root dilatation).

## IMAGING

| CXR | Suggestive of the diagnosis (see Figure 11.3) |
|-----|-----------------------------------------------|
| CT and MRI | Shows size and involvement of branching vessels Can also be used to follow up patients before and after surgery |

## MANAGEMENT

- Surgery should be considered in:
  - Aortic root dilatation of more than 5.5 cm or thoracic aortic dilatation of more than 6 cm in asymptomatic patients.
  - Complications including stroke and spinal ischaemia.
- Endovascular techniques, including covered stenting, are becoming more readily available.

## RARE BUT IMPORTANT CAUSES OF AORTIC DILATATION

### Marfan's syndrome

- A rare genetic disorder leading to connective tissue damage.
- Autosomal-dominant inheritance and spontaneous mutations.
- A variety of features may be present:
  - Skeletal abnormalities
  - Arachnodactyly

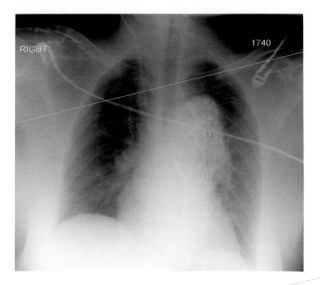

**Figure 11.3** Thoracic aortic aneurysm on a plain AP radiograph. Notice the wide mediastinum and the stent in place in the aortic lumen.

- Lens subluxation
- Aortic and mitral valve regurgitation
- Principle cardiac features:
  - Aortic root dilatation
  - Increased risk of dissection
- Aortic root diameter is monitored and consideration of repair or replacement occurs when diameter reaches a threshold; the European Society of Cardiology recommends intervention with a maximal aortic diameter of ≥5.0 or 4.5 cm if additional risk factors are present.
- Special care is needed during pregnancy when there is an increased risk of rapid expansion and rupture.

## Takayasu's aortitis

- Commonly affects young females of East Asian heritage.
- Large vessel granulomatous vasculitis with associations with other connective tissue disorders.
- The disease causes loss of the elastic layer of the aorta and intimal enlargement and fibrosis.
- Common presentations include teenagers with:
  - Malaise
  - Fever
  - Arthralgia
  - Pleuritic pain

Cardiology and the cardiovascular system

- Aneurysm and stenosis of the aorta and branching vessels can occur:
  - May lead to absent peripheral pulses – the condition is also known as 'pulseless disease' for this reason.
- Treatment focuses on immunosuppression and management of complications as they arise.

## Syphilitic aortitis (rare today)

- Due to spirochaete infection of the tunica media.
- Most commonly during tertiary syphilis.
- Leads to chronic inflammation and weakening of the aortic wall.
- Syphilis should form a differential diagnosis in all patients with ascending aortic dilatation.
- There is no evidence to show that treatment reverses or halts the aortic damage.
- Surgery may be necessary.

# 11.3 AORTIC TRAUMA

- Aortic rupture can result from high-energy trauma.
  - Most commonly chest trauma in high impact vehicle accidents
- The injury most commonly occurs at the junction between the mobile aortic arch and the fixed descending aorta.
- This may be apparent on CXR.
- Commonly the injury is fatal.
- Urgent surgery is necessary but may be contraindicated due to other injuries and predicted poor outcomes.

---

**MICRO-case**

A 45-year-old man attended the ED via ambulance after suddenly experiencing central chest pain. The pain was extremely severe and was not alleviated by painkillers or positional change. The chest pain was described as central, tearing in nature and radiated through to the interscapular region. He felt sweaty, breathless and unwell, and was unusually pale. On initial assessment, he was tachycardic and hypotensive. An ECG revealed a sinus tachycardia and no other abnormalities. He was treated with narcotic analgesics for the pain. While awaiting further investigations he suddenly deteriorated with severe hypotension, which was unresponsive to a fluid challenge. Heart sounds were muffled on auscultation and the jugular vein appeared distended. Cardiac tamponade was suspected; an immediate emergency pericardiocentesis was performed which revealed a haemorrhagic pericardial effusion. An echocardiogram demonstrated a type A aortic dissection extending

*continued...*

*continued...*

into the pericardium. He was sent for urgent surgical repair of the aortic dissection. While recovering on the ward, he was investigated for possible causes of aortic dissection. He had no previous history of hypertension or CVD. He was normally fit and well, a non-smoker and a keen basketball player. He had a pneumothorax at the age of 25. He was of tall stature with a high arch palate and arachnodactyly, and a diagnosis of Marfan's syndrome was made clinically and confirmed by genetic testing. Family members were also tested.

**Points to consider:**

- Marfan's syndrome is an autosomal-dominant condition that can affect the heart, lungs, joints and eyes.
- Aortic dissection can mimic a myocardial infarction.
- All patients admitted with severe chest pain should be examined for radio-radio and radio-femoral delay as aortic dissection may lead to asymmetry in pulses.
- A chest radiograph may reveal widening of the superior mediastinum with proximal aortic dissection.

Cardiology and the cardiovascular system

# A guide to ECG interpretation

## 12.1 ECG INTERPRETATION

It is useful to have a routine method of interpreting ECGs to avoid missing salient features.

> **MICRO-facts**
>
> Large square: 200 ms
> Small square: 40 ms
> Paper speed: 25 mm/s
> Paper voltage: 1 mV = 10 mm
>     When the depolarization wave is moving towards a particular lead, the lead will show a positive deflection.

### RATE

Calculate beats per minute (60–100 bpm)

- Multiply number of QRS complexes in a 10-second strip (standard ECG trace) by 6
- 300 divided by RR interval (number of large squares)

### RHYTHM TO ASSESS

See Chapters 13 and 14 on arrhythmias.

### AXIS

Normal axis is between −30° and +90°.

Right axis deviation

- >+90° indicates right axis deviation, showing a negative deflection in lead I, and a positive one in leads II and III (see Figure 3.4 for cardiac axis diagram).
- **R**ight axis deviation – QRS complexes **R**eaching towards each other in leads I and II.
- Causes include right ventricular hypertrophy, right bundle branch block, left posterior hemiblock, chronic obstructive pulmonary disease, Brugada syndrome, Wolff–Parkinson–White syndrome.

### Left axis deviation

- Between –30° and –90° indicates left axis deviation, showing a positive deflection in lead I and a negative one in leads II and III.
- Left axis deviation – QRS complexes **L**eaving each other in leads I and II.
- Causes include left anterior hemiblock, Wolff–Parkinson–White syndrome and possibly left ventricular hypertrophy.

## P WAVES

- Atrial depolarization.
- P waves may appear to have different morphologies with varying PR intervals, indicating ectopic or multifocal atrial beats.
- A peaked P wave *P pulmonale*: right atrial enlargement (more than three small squares high) (see Figure 12.1).
- A bifid P wave *P mitrale*: left atrial enlargement (more than three small squares wide).

## PR INTERVAL

- 120–200 ms time for depolarization wave to travel from the sinus node to the AV node and through the AV node.
- Measured from the beginning of the P wave to the beginning of the first deflection of the QRS complex.
- Longer than five small squares defines first-degree heart block.
- Shorter than three small squares may indicate Wolff–Parkinson–White syndrome.

## QRS COMPLEX

- <120 ms ventricular depolarization.
- Q is the first negative deflection, R is the first positive deflection and S is the negative deflection after a positive deflection.
- Upper case is used to describe a dominant wave (so an Rs complex is a predominantly positive complex with a small negative deflection afterwards as seen usually in lead V5/V6).

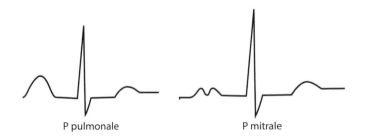

P pulmonale                    P mitrale

**Figure 12.1** P wave morphology.

- Narrow or broad complex:
  - Narrow complex suggests depolarization is through the AV node and down the bundle of His, leading to fast and organized depolarization as in normal physiology.
  - Broad complex in isolation can be a ventricular ectopic.
- If all QRS complexes are broad, consider bundle branch block (which will prolong the time needed to depolarize the ventricles) or at high heart rates consider ventricular tachycardia (see Figures 12.2 and 12.3).

## MICRO-facts

*Left bundle branch block*
Deep S wave in lead V1 (looks like a 'W')
RsR pattern in lead V6 (looks like a 'M')

Note: WiLLiaM

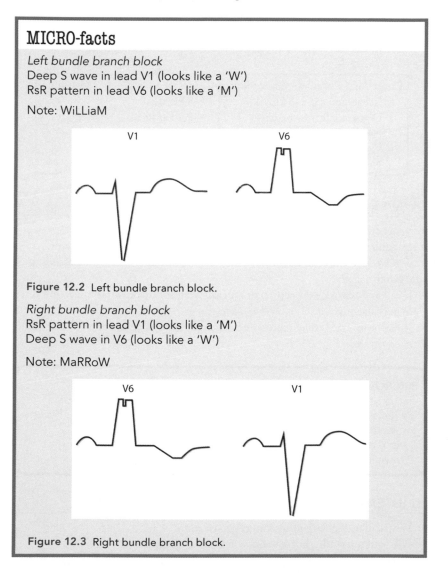

Figure 12.2 Left bundle branch block.

*Right bundle branch block*
RsR pattern in lead V1 (looks like a 'M')
Deep S wave in V6 (looks like a 'W')

Note: MaRRoW

Figure 12.3 Right bundle branch block.

## ST SEGMENT

- Usually on isoelectric line.
- Elevation or depression is usually abnormal.
- Benign early repolarization ('high take-off') is a normal variant seen in people mainly under the age of 50 years and presents with concave ST segment elevation mainly in the anterior precordial leads (may be difficult to differentiate from pathological ST segment elevation).
- If there is left bundle branch block, then it is difficult to comment on ST segment deviation.
- Criteria such as Sgarbossa can be used to assess for myocardial infarction ischaemic changes in the presence of left bundle branch block.

| Causes of ST segment depression: | Causes of ST segment elevation: |
|---|---|
| • Ischaemia, e.g. NSTEMI | • STEMI |
| • Digoxin effect or toxicity | • Pericarditis |
| • Hypokalaemia | • Ventricular aneurysm |
| • Ventricular hypertrophy | • Brugada syndrome |
| • Hyperadrenergic states | |

## T WAVES

- Ventricular repolarization.
- In adults, T wave inversion in V1, III or aVF may be a normal variant.
- T wave inversion can occur normally in aVL but only when the preceding QRS is negative.
- If tall and tented, may represent an early stage of myocardial infarction or hyperkalaemia.
- If flat or inverted, may represent ischaemia, hypokalaemia or a subarachnoid haemorrhage.

> **MICRO-print**
> In the presence of left bundle branch block, the T wave should be deflected in the opposite direction of the last wave in the QRS. This is known as *T wave discordance*.
> In the presence of right bundle branch block, there is commonly T wave inversion in the right precordial leads (V1–V3).

## QT INTERVAL

- Ventricular depolarization and repolarization.
- This will normally shorten as the heart rate increases.

- Correct the length for rate by using Bazett's formula:

$$QTc \text{ (milliseconds)} = \frac{QT \text{ (milliseconds)}}{\sqrt{RR} \text{ (seconds)}}$$

- Although exact figures are debatable, in males QTc is prolonged if >440 ms and in females QTc is prolonged if >460 ms.
- A prolonged QTc interval will predispose to arrhythmias such as torsades de pointes.
- A short QTc (<320 ms) may be suggestive of an inherited channelopathy that predisposes to atrial and ventricular fibrillation and sudden cardiac death.

---

## MICRO-facts

Causes of prolonged QT interval:
- Congenital long QT syndrome
- Low $K^+$, $Mg^{2+}$ or $Ca^{2+}$
- Use of class III anti-arrhythmics such as sotalol and amiodarone
- Use of psychotropic drugs (e.g. citalopram and tricyclic antidepressants)
- Narcotics
- Raised intracranial pressure such as in subarachnoid haemorrhage
- Myotonic dystrophy
- Acute MI

---

### R WAVE PROGRESSION

- Normally, there is a change from a predominantly greater amplitude S wave compared to R wave to a predominantly taller R wave compared to S wave from precordial leads V1–V6 (see Figure 12.4).
- The transition occurs approximately at V2 or V3.

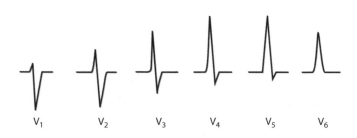

**Figure 12.4** Normal R wave progression.

- The transition zone depends on the orientation of the interventricular septum in the chest (clockwise or counterclockwise cardiac rotation).
- Poor R wave progression may represent an old anterior infarct.

## ADDITIONAL POINTS

*Q waves*
- Defined as a negative deflection *before* an R wave in a QRS complex.
- May be pathological if >25% of accompanying R wave, deeper than two small squares and wider than one small square.
- May be a normal variant even with these characteristics in lead III.
- Pathological Q waves represent electrical silence or 'dead myocardium'.

*J waves (Osborn wave)*
- A rounded wave that follows the R wave in the QRS complex and indicates hypothermia.

*U wave*
- A rounded wave that follows the T wave and may indicate hypokalaemia.

Summary of approach
- Rate and rhythm
- Axis: normal, left or right
- P waves: absent or present
- PR interval: long, short or normal
- QRS complex: narrow or broad
- ST segment: isoelectric, elevated or depressed
- T waves: upright or inverted
- QT interval: short, long or normal
- R wave progression
- Additional waves

---

**MICRO-print**
**Paediatric ECG**

In utero, the pulmonary circulation is very high resistance compared to the systemic circulation. To push blood through this, the RV is thicker and larger than the LV. This is demonstrable on an ECG as a pattern of RV dominance at birth similar to RV hypertrophy: right axis deviation, tall R waves in right precordial leads (V1–V3) and upright T waves in right precordial leads (V1–V3).

With the first few breaths, there is a fall in intrathoracic pressure in the neonate and a subsequent decrease in pulmonary vascular resistance, and an increase in systemic vascular resistance that within the first month of life results in a larger and thicker LV compared to RV.

*continued...*

*continued...*

Normally, sometime during the first week of life the upright T waves in V1–V3 on a neonatal ECG will become inverted, resulting in the typical 'juvenile T wave inversion pattern' that may persist variably into adolescence. As a child ages, the T waves will become upright first in V3 and then V2. Many adults will demonstrate ongoing T wave inversion in V1.

Resting heart rates and conduction intervals differ in children and vary with age.

Cardiology and the cardiovascular system

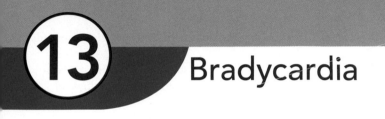

# 13 Bradycardia

## 13.1 SINUS NODE-RELATED BRADYCARDIA

### SINUS BRADYCARDIA

Cardiac causes

- Increased vagal tone, e.g. in athletes
- Drug induced, e.g. verapamil, diltiazem, beta-blockers
- Intrinsic disease of the sinus node:
    - Ischaemia: supplied by the right coronary artery in up to 70% of the population, and by the left circumflex artery in up to 30%
    - Fibrosis secondary to age, ischaemia, cardiomyopathy, congenital dysfunction or myotonic dystrophy
- Acute MI (especially inferior MI)

Non-cardiac causes

- Neurally mediated via the Bezold–Jarisch reflex:
    - Carotid sinus syndrome
    - Neurocardiogenic syncope
- Hypothyroidism
- Hypothermia
- Raised intracranial pressure (as part of Cushing's triad)
- Severe cholestatic jaundice and hepatitis
- Infections, e.g. typhoid leading to relative bradycardia

### SINUS NODE DYSFUNCTION

- Arrhythmias caused by dysfunction of the sinus node

> **MICRO-facts**
>
> Sinus node dysfunction with symptoms is known as sick sinus syndrome. Symptoms may include dizziness, fatigue, palpitations or collapse.

## Sinus pause

- Failure of electrical discharge from the sinus node lasting at least 2 seconds but followed by a sinus beat
- ECG: failure of the P wave to appear when expected and reappearance at a later point followed by a QRS complex; the pause is not a multiple of the P–P interval

## Sinus arrest

- Failure of electrical discharge from the sinus node lasting at least 2 seconds during which time a junctional escape beat will result in ventricular depolarization
- ECG: failure of the P wave to appear when expected; with appearance of a QRS complex called a junctional escape beat

## Sinus exit block

- Sinus node discharges normally but this is not transmitted to the atria.
- Three degrees exist.
- ECG: failure of the P wave to appear when expected; the resulting pause between the P waves is a multiple of the P–P interval.

## Tachy brady syndrome

- A form of sick sinus syndrome in which bradycardias coexist with paroxysmal supraventricular tachycardias

---

**MICRO-print**

An implantable loop ECG recorder is a small device inserted in a subcutaneous pocket that can stay in place for prolonged periods of time and record a single ECG lead to establish evidence for cardiac arrhythmia. It may be activated to record a rhythm on its own by preset parameters or be activated by the patient when symptoms occur.

---

### MANAGEMENT

- Treat the patient as per the ALS bradycardia algorithm (see Figure 13.4).

# 13.2 HEART BLOCK (SEE FIGURE 13.1)

## ATRIOVENTRICULAR (AV) BLOCK (SEE FIGURE 13.2)

### Cardiac causes

- Ischaemic heart disease or acute MI (especially inferior MI)
- Drugs: beta-blockers, rate-limiting calcium channel blockers and other anti-arrhythmics
- Conduction system fibrosis (Lev's disease and Lenegre's disease)

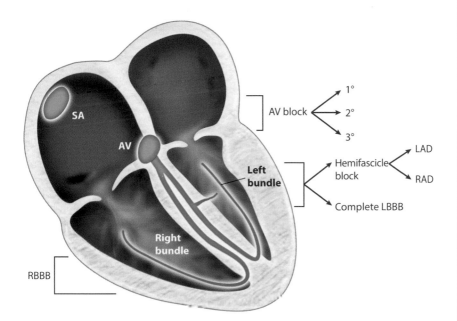

**Figure 13.1** Heart block summary.

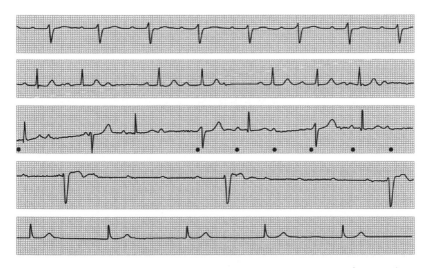

**Figure 13.2** ECG of AV block. A: First-degree heart block. B: Mobitz type I second-degree heart block. C: Mobitz type II second-degree heart block with 2:1 block and narrow complex escape rhythm; note the red dots under the regular P waves and the negative deflection of the escape QRS beats. D: Third-degree heart block; note the regularity of the P waves and the QRS complex and their complete lack of association. E: Third-degree heart block; note the narrow complex bradycardia and the absence of P waves suggests AF with complete heart block.

- Calcific aortic valve stenosis or root abscess (infective endocarditis)
- Cardiomyopathy
- Cardiac surgery or catheter ablation
- Autoimmune disease (maternal systemic lupus erythematosus with foetal complete heart block)
- Muscular dystrophy (especially myotonic dystrophy)

### Non-cardiac causes

- Hypothyroidism
- Hypothermia

### First degree

- Prolongation of the PR interval (>200 ms) due to delayed conduction from the atria through the AV node

### Second degree

- *Mobitz type I (Wenckebach):* sequential prolongation of the PR interval until there is a dropped QRS complex resulting in an irregular R–R interval (tends to be an abnormality of the AV node).
- *Mobitz type II:* PR interval is constant but there is a dropped QRS complex every few beats, giving, for example a 2:1 or 3:1 block (tends to be an abnormality in the bundle of His).

### Third degree

- Complete dissociation between the atrial and ventricular contraction electrically and functionally.
- P waves are not conducted down to the ventricles.
- Both P waves and QRS complexes occur at regular intervals but with no association between the two (P–P is constant and R–R is constant).
- The P wave rate is faster than the QRS complex rate.
- *Narrow complex third-degree heart block:* the pacemaker resulting in ventricular contractions is just below the AV node or in the bundle of His.
- *Broad complex third-degree heart block:* the pacemaker is beyond the bundle of His, resulting in a less-well conducted contraction and therefore a broad complex QRS.

  *NB:* This is a dangerous morphology in third-degree heart block and merits immediate pacing.

---

## MICRO-facts

In a Stokes–Adam attack, a patient typically turns pale and collapses to the ground. They will flush and recover within seconds. This is typically caused by a bradyarrhythmia such as complete heart block leading to decreased cardiac output and reduced cerebral perfusion.

---

Cardiology and the cardiovascular system

# 13.3 BUNDLE BRANCH BLOCK

## RIGHT BUNDLE BRANCH BLOCK (RBBB)

- A single right bundle derives from the bundle of His and supplies Purkinje fibres to the right ventricle.
- See Figure 12.3 for ECG pattern.

## LEFT BUNDLE BRANCH BLOCK (LBBB)

- A posterior and an anterior fascicle derive from the bundle of His and supply Purkinje fibres to the left ventricle.
- See Figure 12.2 for ECG pattern.
- Right axis deviation results from isolated left posterior fascicle block.
- Left axis deviation results from isolated left anterior fascicle block.

## BIFASCICULAR BLOCK

- RBBB with left anterior fascicle hemiblock (left axis deviation)
- RBBB with left posterior fascicle hemiblock (right axis deviation)
- LBBB alone

## TRIFASCICULAR BLOCK

- Trifascicular block is a misnomer: when all three fascicles are blocked, this results in complete (third-degree) AV block.
- However, it is often used to refer to bifascicular block and first-degree AV block (see Figure 13.3).

|  | CARDIAC | NON-CARDIAC |
|---|---|---|
| Causes of RBBB | Acute MI<br>Cardiomyopathy<br>Conduction system fibrosis<br>Atrial septal defect<br>Pulmonary stenosis | Cor pulmonale<br>PE<br>Pulmonary<br>  hypertension |
| Causes of LBBB | Acute MI<br>Ischaemic heart disease<br>Cardiomyopathy<br>Aortic stenosis | Hypertension |

### MANAGEMENT

- In a haemodynamically stable patient, first-degree and Mobitz type I second-degree AV block and bundle branch block are stable rhythms.

Cardiology and the cardiovascular system

Cardiology and the cardiovascular system

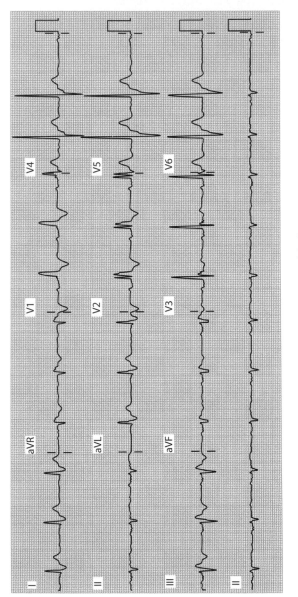

Figure 13.3 'Trifascicular block'; RBBB, left axis deviation and first-degree AV block.

- The majority may never progress to higher degrees of block, but in some cases there is a tendency to progress to complete heart block.
- Progression is slow, over years depending on the aetiology.
- In haemodynamic instability, follow the management plan as per ALS guidelines for bradycardia (see Figure 13.4).

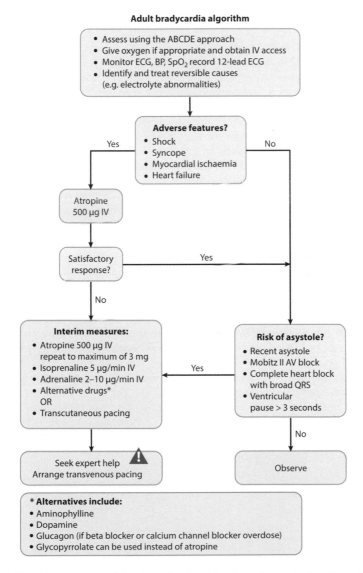

**Adult bradycardia algorithm**

- Assess using the ABCDE approach
- Give oxygen if appropriate and obtain IV access
- Monitor ECG, BP, SpO₂ record 12-lead ECG
- Identify and treat reversible causes (e.g. electrolyte abnormalities)

**Adverse features?**
- Shock
- Syncope
- Myocardial ischaemia
- Heart failure

Yes → Atropine 500 μg IV

No →

Satisfactory response? — Yes →

No ↓

**Interim measures:**
- Atropine 500 μg IV repeat to maximum of 3 mg
- Isoprenaline 5 μg/min IV
- Adrenaline 2–10 μg/min IV
- Alternative drugs*
  OR
- Transcutaneous pacing

Yes ←

**Risk of asystole?**
- Recent asystole
- Mobitz II AV block
- Complete heart block with broad QRS
- Ventricular pause > 3 seconds

No ↓

Seek expert help
Arrange transvenous pacing

Observe

**\* Alternatives include:**
- Aminophylline
- Dopamine
- Glucagon (if beta blocker or calcium channel blocker overdose)
- Glycopyrrolate can be used instead of atropine

**Figure 13.4** Management of bradycardia algorithm from Resuscitation Council. (From Peri-arrest Arrhythmias. With permission.)

**MICRO-case**

A 61-year-old woman called 999 because she experienced sudden onset of left-sided chest pain along with dizziness. Within 10 minutes, the paramedics found her in a collapsed state at home. On examination, she was clammy, her pulse was thready at 45 bpm and her blood pressure was 82/42 mmHg. An ECG revealed 2 mm ST depression and T wave inversion in leads II, III, aVF with sinus bradycardia. The attending physician made a diagnosis of acute inferior NSTEMI complicated by bradycardia. He immediately obtained intravenous access and sent off venous samples for investigations including cardiac enzymes and electrolytes. Given her clinically shocked state, the patient was given intravenous atropine 500 μg twice with good effect. She was treated for an acute coronary syndrome and moved to the coronary care unit where she was placed on continuous cardiac monitoring. It was later noted that the heart rhythm showed intermittent Wenckebach block, which was well tolerated with no haemodynamic effect. The abnormality resolved over a further 24 hours. She was very anxious and worried that she would need a permanent pacemaker. Her cardiologist explained to her that sometimes patients who have had an inferior infarction develop transient heart block but this rarely is persistent and pacemakers are usually not necessary. She was discharged home well after angiography and stent insertion in the right coronary artery.

**Points to consider:**

- Inferior myocardial infarctions affect the vagal-fibre rich inferior heart surface so may cause sinus bradycardia due to increased vagotonic effect.
- The onset of higher degree AV block in acute inferior MI is most likely due to ischaemia of the AV node; the right coronary artery is responsible for blood supply to the AV node in the majority of individuals.
- Most patients with bradycardia from acute inferior MI do not require permanent pacemakers.
- For patients presenting with bradycardia, it is important to follow the ALS algorithm.

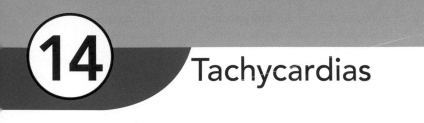

# 14 Tachycardias

## 14.1 NARROW COMPLEX TACHYCARDIA (SEE FIGURE 14.1)

### SINUS TACHYCARDIA

#### CAUSES

- Sinus tachycardia may be a physiological response to maintain cardiac output and therefore organ perfusion when there is a fall in peripheral vascular resistance or stroke volume.
- This can be explained by understanding the determinants of cardiac output and blood pressure as per the equations below:

  Cardiac output (CO) = stroke volume (SV) × heart rate (HR)

  Blood pressure (BP) = CO × peripheral vascular resistance (PVR).

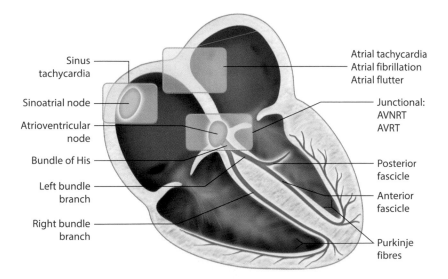

**Figure 14.1** Summary of narrow complex tachycardia.

- Some examples of when this compensatory mechanism occurs:
  - Pulmonary embolism (most common ECG feature is sinus tachycardia)
  - Infection with sepsis
  - Fever
  - Dehydration or blood loss
  - Heart failure
  - Anaphylaxis
  - Pregnancy to facilitate the increased cardiac output necessary to grow the foetus
  - Iron deficiency anaemia
- Increase in sympathetic drive:
  - Anxiety
  - Hyperthyroidism
  - Pain
  - Drugs, e.g. bronchodilators, aminophyllines

### ECG FEATURES

- Sinus rhythm with a rate >100 bpm and usually <150 bpm

## ATRIAL TACHYCARDIA

### MECHANISM

- Focus of pacing is elsewhere in the atria, not at the sinoatrial node.
- Majority originate from the right atrium.

### ECG FEATURES

- May demonstrate abnormal P wave morphology.
- *Multifocal atrial tachycardia* is a specific form of atrial tachycardia character-ized by at least three different P wave morphologies and varying PR interval lengths demonstrating multiple foci of atrial depolarization conducting to the AV node.
- Often degenerates to AF over time.

### TREATMENT

- Reversal of precipitating factors including infection.
- Use of rate-limiting agents that delay AV nodal conduction such as beta-blockers or rate-limiting calcium channel blockers.
- Amiodarone is very effective for multifocal atrial tachycardia.

> **MICRO-facts**
>
> Causes of irregular narrow complex tachycardia:
> - Atrial fibrillation.
> - Atrial flutter with variable block.
> - Multifocal atrial tachycardia that is usually associated with chronic obstructive pulmonary disease, sepsis or drug toxicity such as with digoxin or theophylline. The rhythm strip will show a varying R–R interval. The atria contract so there is no increase in the risk of thromboembolism.

## ATRIAL FIBRILLATION

### MECHANISM

- Uncoordinated contraction of the atrial myocytes with spontaneous depolarization resulting in a tachycardia and in a variability in conduction to the ventricles via the AV node.
- The rate is limited by the speed of conduction through the AV node – known as the Wenckebach point (usually 180–220 bpm).

### CAUSES

- The basic physiological trigger is atrial dilatation.
- Any cause of atrial stretch will precipitate AF.

#### Cardiac causes

- Ageing degeneration (10% of 80-year-olds)
- Ischaemic heart disease usually associated with heart failure
- Heart failure
- Valvular heart disease, especially mitral valve disease
- Hypertension (the most common association)

#### Non-cardiac causes

- Pulmonary embolism
- Pneumonia
- Other sources of sepsis
- Alcohol
- Hyperthyroidism
- Post-operative

### ECG FEATURES

- Irregularly irregular R–R interval due to variable conduction down the AV node
- No discernible P waves
- P waves replaced by chaotic electrical baseline: may be *fine* or *coarse*

## MICRO-facts

*Paroxysmal* AF may be recurrent and terminates spontaneously in less than 7 days.

*Persistent* AF is present continuously for at least 7 days or only terminates with chemical or electrical cardioversion.

*Permanent* AF has either been resistant to cardioversion or has not been cardioverted.

### SYMPTOMS AND SIGNS

### SYMPTOMS

- Palpitations
- Chest pain in those with coronary artery disease (myocardial blood flow only occurs in diastole so tachycardia will reduce diastolic time, thereby exacerbating myocardial insufficiency)
- Dizziness/syncope (caused by the drop in blood pressure from loss of synchronized atrial systole)
- Breathlessness and orthopnoea (symptoms of impaired left ventricular filling precipitated by loss of atrial synchronous contraction)

### SIGNS

- Irregularly irregular pulse
- Absence of 'a' wave in the JVP
- Signs of heart failure and peripheral hypoperfusion

### TREATMENT

- There is a need to manage **both** the AF itself and the risk of atrial thrombus and subsequent cerebrovascular accidents (see Figure 14.2).

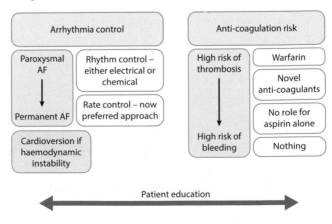

Figure 14.2 AF treatment summary.

> **MICRO-print**
>
> In atrial fibrillation, the lack of synchronization between atrial myocytes means that the atria do not contract effectively. There is no atrial 'kick' at the end of diastole, reducing ventricular filling and resultant cardiac output by at least 10%. Note that ventricular filling will already be reduced due to shortening of diastole in the presence of a tachycardia. Therefore, atrial fibrillation with a fast ventricular response may have significant haemodynamic effects, especially in a heart with already reduced ejection fraction, and those depending on active atrial transport – as in left ventricular hypertrophy.
>
> Uncoordinated atrial contraction causes intra-atrial turbulence and increased risk of spontaneous thrombus formation. Embolic occlusion of systemic arteries can cause strokes, mesenteric ischaemia or peripheral limb ischaemia.

### Rhythm control

*Patient group*

- Now offered only in selected patients as rate control is the predominant strategy.
- Necessary in those with haemodynamic instability as a priority over thrombosis risk.
- In addition, it is useful in the following patients with AF:
  - Secondary to a treated or corrected precipitant
  - New-onset AF with a history consistent with specific and recent onset heart failure caused primarily by AF (very rare – in most cases, AF is secondary to CCF)

### Thrombosis risk management for electrical rhythm control

- Heparin cover if within 48 hours of AF onset.
- Three weeks of preceding anti-coagulation followed by at least 4 weeks of anti-coagulation if AF onset is greater than 48 hours or unknown.
- If a trans-oesophageal echocardiogram has shown no intracardiac thrombus, it may be safe to cardiovert without anti-coagulation.

### Methods

- Electrical cardioversion under sedation or general anaesthetic by synchronizing with R waves (an accidental unsynchronized cardiac shock during a T wave may lead to ventricular fibrillation).
- Chemical cardioversion under cardiac monitoring:
  - Amiodarone for patients with structural heart disease
  - Flecainide for patients without structural heart disease
- Catheter ablation may be an effective elective treatment in a select group of patients.

Cardiology and the cardiovascular system

> **MICRO-print**
> The term 'structural heart disease' includes ventricular dysfunction, ischaemic heart disease, valvular heart disease or defects in cardiac anatomy. Be very wary of giving amiodarone to any patient already on sotalol for a rate control strategy as the combination of these agents may prolong QTc and predispose to arrhythmias.

Rate control

| First line | Beta-blocker or calcium channel blocker |
|------------|------------------------------------------|
| Second line | Add on digoxin<br>NB: Digoxin alone is effective only in sedentary patients<br>Optimal heart rate control usually requires a combination of beta-blocker and digoxin – never use beta-blockers with a rate-limiting calcium channel blocker |

> **MICRO-reference**
> National Institute for Health and Care Excellence. Atrial fibrillation. NICE guidelines [CG180]. London: National Institute for Health and Care Excellence, 2014.

Long-term anti-coagulation
- Risk stratification tools used to quantify the risk of thrombosis and bleeding may help direct anti-coagulation decisions.
- Patients with paroxysmal AF have a similar risk of ischaemic stroke as those with permanent AF, and therefore merit equal consideration for long-term anti-coagulation.
- Example of thrombosis risk-determining tool: $CHA_2DS_2VASc$.
- Example of bleeding risk-determining tool: HAS-BLED.
- Scores will correlate with observed stroke and bleeding risks in studied populations.
- Some factors will unfortunately contribute to both thrombosis and bleeding risk.
- *A $CHA_2DS_2VASc$ score of zero corresponds to a stroke risk of 0.78% per year – do not offer these patients anti-coagulation.*
- *A $CHA_2DS_2VASc$ score of 1 corresponds to a stroke risk of 2% per year – consider anti-coagulation only in men with this score.*
- *Anti-coagulation should be considered for all patients with a $CHA_2DS_2VASc$ score of 2 or more while taking into account the bleeding risk.*

- Aspirin alone is no longer recommended for the prevention of stroke in patients with AF.
- Novel oral anti-coagulants such as rivaroxaban should be considered in a subset of patients.

| THROMBOSIS | | BLEEDING | |
|---|---|---|---|
| C | Congestive heart failure | H | Hypertension |
| H | Hypertension | A (1 or 2 pts) | Abnormal renal/liver function |
| A (2 pts) | Age ≥75 | S | Previous stroke |
| D | Diabetes mellitus | B | Bleeding |
| S (2 pts) | Previous stroke/TIA | L | Labile INR |
| V | Vascular disease | E | Elderly |
| A | Age 65–74 | D (1 or 2 pts) | Alcohol or drugs (NSAIDs, anti-platelet) |
| Sc | Sex category female | | |
| | *9 points total* | | *9 points total* |

---

**MICRO-references**

Pisters R, Lane DA, Nieuwlaat R, et al. A novel user-friendly score (HAS-BLED) to assess one-year risk of major bleeding in atrial fibrillation patients: the Euro Heart Survey. *Chest* 2010; 138(5): 1093–1100.

Lip GY, Nieuwlaat R, Pisters R, et al. Refining clinical risk stratification for predicting stroke and thromboembolism in atrial fibrillation using a novel risk factor-based approach: the Euro Heart Survey on atrial fibrillation. *Chest* 2010; 137: 263–272.

---

**MICRO-facts**

Atrial fibrillation not only predisposes to ischaemic strokes but those resultant strokes are worse than strokes in patients without atrial fibrillation. Atrial fibrillation is associated with greater volume strokes, increased mortality rates and worse neurological impairment.

Cardiology and the cardiovascular system

| DECISION TO ANTI-COAGULATE ACCORDING TO NICE 2014 GUIDELINES | | |
|---|---|---|
| CHA$_2$DS$_2$VASc Score 0 | CHA$_2$DS$_2$VASc Score 1 | CHA$_2$DS$_2$VASc Score 2 or more |
| Annual risk of stroke 0.78% | Annual risk of stroke is 2% | Annual risk of stroke is 3.7% or more |
| Do not offer anti-coagulation | In women offer no anti-coagulation In men consider anti-coagulation | Offer anti-coagulation once bleeding risk has been assessed |

## ATRIAL FLUTTER

### MECHANISM

- A macro re-entry supraventricular tachycardia
- Caused by a re-entrant mechanism:
  - *Type I* located near the tricuspid annulus and through the tricuspid-cavo isthmus in the right atrium
  - *Type II* originate in other parts of the right atrium or the left atrium

### CAUSES AND SYMPTOMS

- Are similar to those of AF (see above)

### ECG FEATURES

- Type I atrial flutter tends to have atrial rates between 240 and 340 bpm.
- Type II atrial flutter tends to have atrial rates between 340 and 440 bpm.
- The AV node will conduct the impulse down to the ventricles, but the Wenckebach point (see above) means there is always 2:1 block or a 3:1 block with a resulting slower regular ventricular rhythm (see Figure 14.3).
- 1:1 conduction occurs down an accessory pathway and may lead to ventricular fibrillation and sudden death.
- P waves are absent, atrial activity is seen as a 'saw-tooth' baseline with identical *flutter* waves.
- Flutter waves may not be distinguishable if the rhythm is fast; slowing down the rhythm (by using vago-tonic reflexes) may reveal underlying flutter waves.

### MANAGEMENT

- Consider pharmacological rate control with agents that delay AV nodal conduction such as digoxin, verapamil, diltiazem or beta-blockers (usually requiring large doses and combinations).
- Consider synchronized electrical cardioversion under sedation or general anaesthetic using lower energy thresholds than those for AF.

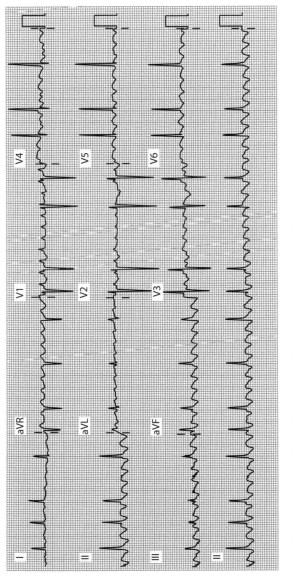

**Figure 14.3** Atrial flutter with variable block; note the flutter waves and saw-tooth pattern.

Cardiology and the cardiovascular system

- Pharmacological cardioversion works well in patients with atrial flutter.
- Consider catheter ablation of the macro re-entry pathway; the resultant scar tissue will stop conduction through the pathway.
- Thromboembolic risk is similar to that in AF and must be managed accordingly.

> ## MICRO-facts
>
> Macro re-entrant tachycardias are caused by extensive areas of the cardiac atria that provide a circuit through which an impulse will propel and re-activate already activated tissue, causing a loop circuit and therefore a self-propagating tachycardia. An example is atrial flutter. This is different from a micro re-entry tachycardia that arises from a more focal area of the myocardium.

## JUNCTIONAL TACHYCARDIA

### MECHANISM

- Regular, narrow complex paroxysmal tachycardias that arise from the region in or near the AV node due to re-entry circuits.
- Common as paroxysmal SVTs in young people with no structural heart disease.
- *AV nodal re-entry tachycardia* (AVNRT) occurs due to an additional path *within* the AV node.
- *AV re-entry tachycardia* (AVRT) occurs due to an additional path *near* the AV node.

### SYMPTOMS

- Usually occurs in paroxysmal episodes.
- Regular, fast palpitations with sudden onset and offset.
- May be exacerbated by sympathomimetic agents like caffeine or drugs.
- Symptoms of dizziness, syncope or chest pain due to haemodynamic compromise may occur.

### ECG

- Usually rate between 140 and 280 bpm.
- Regular, narrow complex tachycardia.
- As atrial conduction may be retrograde, with impulses travelling upwards, P waves may be inverted in the inferior leads (II, III, aVF).
- P waves may be hidden in the QRS complex (common in slow–fast AVNRT).
- P waves may occur after the QRS complex (common in fast–slow AVNRT).

## MICRO-print

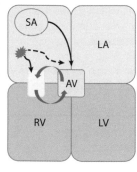

### AVRT mechanism

*Orthodromic conduction – down the AV node and up the accessory bundle*

Sinus nodal impulse is propagated down the AV node, which will become temporarily refractory to further impulses. However, if an ectopic atrial beat should reach the AV node before the sinus impulse, it may then propagate down this node and back up to the atria through the accessory pathway (as this may not be refractory at this time unlike the AV node). A loop circuit is formed resulting in tachycardia.

The circuit cycles clockwise.

*Antidromic conduction – down the accessory bundle and up the AV node (rarer)*

Sinus nodal impulse is propagated down the AV node, which will temporarily become refractory to further impulses. If an ectopic atrial beat should result in an impulse at this time, it will not be able to travel down the AV node but will be able to travel down an accessory pathway. Once it has done so, the AV node may have stopped being refractory, at which point the impulse can travel inappropriately up the AV node and back to the atria, from where it will carry down the accessory pathway again. This forms a loop tachycardia.

The circuit cycles anticlockwise.

## MICRO-print

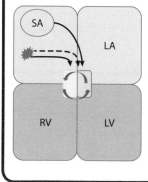

### AV nodal re-entry tachycardia (AVNRT) mechanism

There are two pathways in the AV node:

- *Slow conduction pathway* with a short refractory period
- *Fast conduction pathway* with a long refractory period

Usually, the sinus nodal impulse travels down both circuits simultaneously and then down the bundle of His. However, if an atrial

*continued...*

Cardiology and the cardiovascular system

*continued...*

ectopic beat develops during this time, it may find the fast pathway still in a refractory period, during which time it will travel down the slow pathway. By this time, the fast pathway may have come out of its refractory period, allowing the impulse to travel back up, activate the atria retrogradely and initiate a tachycardia circuit. This is *slow–fast* AVNRT and is commoner than *fast–slow* AVNRT in which anterograde conduction is through the fast pathway and retrograde conduction to the atria is via the slow pathway.

### MANAGEMENT

- Treat as per the regular narrow QRS complex section of the ALS tachyarrhythmia algorithm shown below (see Figure 14.6).
- Note that the options for vagal manoeuvres include the Valsalva manoeuvre, carotid sinus massage and facial immersion in cold water.
- Cardiac ablation therapy may be appropriate in a select group of patients.

Wolff–Parkinson–White syndrome (WPW syndrome)

- A form of AVRT in which the accessory pathway is the **bundle of Kent**.
- This pathway conducts some of the sinus impulse to the ventricles, leading to early depolarization of a part of the ventricle.
- This is seen on the ECG as slurring of the upstroke of the QRS complex (delta wave) and a short PR interval (see Figure 14.4).
- In antidromic activation, the activation of the ventricles is primarily through the bundle of Kent, resulting in depolarization of the ventricles that is not through the bundle of His and therefore a broad complex tachycardia.
- Patients who develop AF will present with an irregular broad complex tachycardia on an ECG, as atrial activity is conducted down the accessory pathway.
- In AF, the accessory pathway may have a shorter refractory period than the AV node and conduct very high rates down to the ventricles resulting in a risk of ventricular fibrillation.

## MICRO-facts

Verapamil, digoxin and adenosine may facilitate the abnormally fast conduction down the accessory pathway and are therefore contraindicated in patients with AF and WPW syndrome.

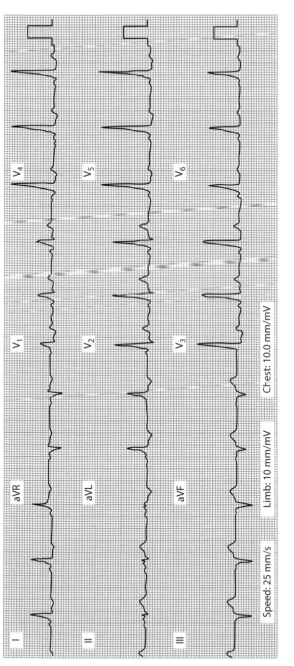

Figure 14.4 WPW ECG. Note the characteristic presence of a delta wave and the short PR interval.

Cardiology and the cardiovascular system

## 14.2 BROAD COMPLEX TACHYCARDIAS

### CAUSES

- Electrolyte abnormalities
- Ischaemic heart disease
- Infective myocarditis
- Cardiomyopathies: infiltrative, inflammatory
- Cardiac channelopathies
- Structural heart conditions such as tetralogy of Fallot

### SYMPTOMS

- May be asymptomatic if haemodynamically stable ventricular tachycardia (VT).
- Symptoms of palpitations, breathlessness, dizziness or collapse may herald haemodynamically unstable VT or ventricular fibrillation, which require immediate direct current cardioversion.

---

**MICRO-print**

**Cardiac channelopathies**

*Congenital long QT syndrome*

- Inherited usually in an autosomal-dominant manner (Romano-Ward syndrome), less commonly in an autosomal-recessive manner (Jervell and Lange-Nielsen syndrome, also associated with congenital high tone deafness).
- Characterized by prolonged ventricular repolarization.
- Arrythmias such as torsades de pointes are usually precipitated by an adrenergic surge, e.g. exercise or emotion.
- Treatment is with beta-blockers or ICD insertion.

*Brugada syndrome*

- Autosomal-dominant inheritance pattern.
- More common in young Southeast Asian males.
- Commonly seen in patients with mutations in *SCN5A*, a gene coding for sodium ion channels in cell membranes.
- RBBB morphology with cove-shaped ST segment elevation in leads V1–V3.
- Different variants exist.
- Risk of ventricular fibrillation necessitates treatment with insertion of an ICD.

*Catecholaminergic polymorphic ventricular tachycardia (CPVT)*

- Genetic abnormality: may be inherited in either an autosomal-dominant or autosomal-recessive pattern.

*continued...*

*continued...*

- Ventricular arrhythmia is precipitated by sympathetic overdrive such as during exercise or intense emotional situations.
- 12-lead ECG may be normal but exercise testing may induce bidirectional VT.

*Arrhythmogenic right ventricular cardiomyopathy (ARVC)*

- Genetic abnormality usually inherited in an autosomal-dominant pattern and associated with fatty infiltration of the right ventricle.
- Arrhythmia originates from the right ventricular outflow tract.
- The ECG may show a characteristic epsilon wave (a positive deflection at the end of a QRS complex).

## MICRO-facts

Ajmaline is an anti-arrhythmic agent that in normal people would produce only a slight widening of the QRS complex. It is used as a provocation test in patients with suspected Brugada syndrome as it will bring on the typical ECG appearance of Brugada in these patients. Changes include ST elevation in leads V1, V2, V3 with or without a pattern of right bundle branch block.

## TYPES AND ECG

### Monomorphic ventricular tachycardia

- Five or more consecutive regular broad complexes at a rate of >100 bpm with constant QRS morphology.
- Non-sustained VT (NSVT) lasts at least five beats but less than 30 seconds (incidence of up to 4%).
- Sustained VT lasts longer than 30 seconds.
- NSVT in the presence of structural heart disease is a bigger risk factor for VT and ventricular fibrillation.
- With pulse, treat as per the broad QRS section of the ALS tachyarrhythmia algorithm shown below (see Figure 14.6), remembering that a regular broad complex tachycardia is VT until proven otherwise if there is a diagnostic uncertainty.

## MICRO-facts

For pulseless VT, refer to the cardiac arrest section (see p. 189)

SVT with aberrancy

- SVT with bundle branch block or pre-excitation through an accessory pathway, e.g. irregular broad complex tachycardia may result from AF with WPW syndrome.
- ECG appears to be a regular or irregular broad complex tachycardia.
- May respond to the regular management of an SVT.
- It is important to differentiate it from VT as the treatment of VT is very different.

> ## MICRO-facts
>
> On a 12-lead ECG, the following features indicate that the arrhythmia is more likely VT than SVT with aberrancy (or use the Brugada criteria):
>
> - Concordant QRS direction in chest leads (all positive or all negative)
> - Marked left axis deviation
> - AV dissociation
> - Capture beat (occasional narrow complex QRS as a P wave is captured by the AV node)
> - Fusion beat (an abnormal QRS complex from the fusion of a capture and a ventricular beat)
>
> If there is any diagnostic doubt assume the trace is VT. In patients with a history of ischaemic heart disease, a broad complex tachycardia is nearly always VT.

Polymorphic ventricular tachycardia

- Regular broad complex tachycardia with beat-to-beat variation in morphology.
- *Torsades de pointes* is a specific example:
  - Characteristic ECG (see Figure 14.5): twisting of the QRS complexes with a cyclical change in the axis.
  - Occurs in the presence of long QT syndrome.
  - Treatment is with IV magnesium if haemodynamically stable (see Figure 14.6).

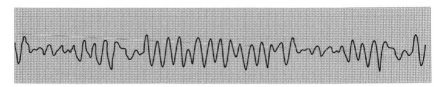

**Figure 14.5** ECG of VT.

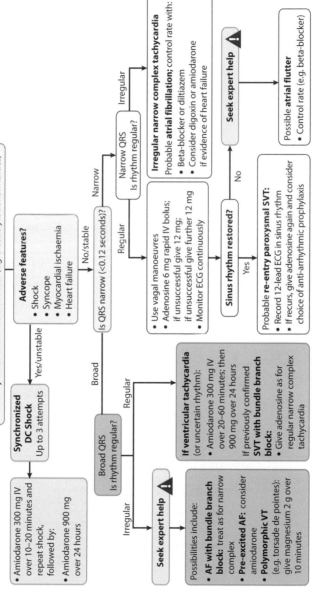

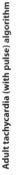

**Figure 14.6** Tachycardia algorithm. Resuscitation Council algorithm for management of tachycardias. (Reproduced with permission.)

Cardiology and the cardiovascular system

# 14.3 CARDIAC ARREST RHYTHMS

- The four rhythms below result in a loss of cardiac output, and it is important to follow the cardiac arrest algorithm (see Figure 14.7) in their treatment.
- Asystole and pulseless electrical activity are not shockable rhythms.
- Pulseless VT and ventricular fibrillation are shockable rhythms.

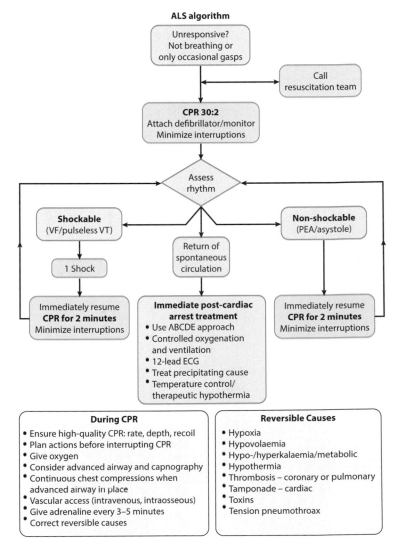

**Figure 14.7** Resuscitation Council UK Advanced Life Support cardiac arrest algorithm. (From Advanced Adult Life Support by the Resuscitation Council. Reproduced with permission.)

Cardiology and the cardiovascular system

## ASYSTOLE

- Lack of electrical activity in the heart resulting in a loss of cardiac output (see Figure 14.8).

## PULSELESS ELECTRICAL ACTIVITY (PEA)

- Electrical activity is present in the heart but there is a loss of cardiac output with no pulse present (use a central artery such as the carotid or the femoral artery to detect a pulse).

## PULSELESS VT

- VT is present with loss of cardiac output.

## VENTRICULAR FIBRILLATION (VF)

- Irregular broad complex tachycardia with variable morphology that invariably results in a loss of cardiac output (see Figure 14.9).

---

**MICRO-facts**

*What is the difference between synchronized and unsynchronized direct current shock?*

An unsynchronized mechanism delivers a shock at any time in the cardiac cycle, whereas a synchronized one will trigger the shock to be delivered on the R wave of the QRS complex to avoid delivering a shock on top of a T wave. Attempted depolarization of the ventricles during repolarization may precipitate VF. Synchronized shocks are used when there is distinguishable T wave activity. High-energy unsynchronized shocks may be used for VF or pulseless VT.

---

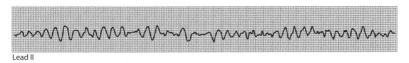

II

**Figure 14.8** ECG of asystole.

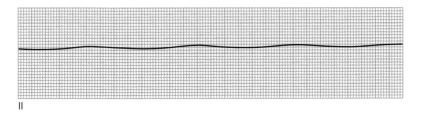

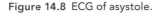
Lead II

**Figure 14.9** ECG of VF.

Cardiology and the cardiovascular system

**MICRO-case**

A 65-year-old woman with a background history of ischaemic heart disease, controlled hypertension and chronic obstructive pulmonary disease (COPD) presented to the emergency department with a 1-month history of intermittent palpitations worse over the past 24 hours. She denied chest pain. On examination, she had a fast irregularly irregular heart rate of 130 beats per minute with no overt signs of heart failure or hypotension. Her drug history comprised a seretide inhaler, ramipril, aspirin, simvastatin and a GTN spray as required. She was an active woman fond of hiking. An ECG displayed AF with a fast ventricular response and a plain chest radiograph was unremarkable. She had normal U&Es, TFTs and urine dipstick. The clinicians found no evidence of underlying myocardial infarction, infection or pulmonary embolism. Given that she was haemodynamically stable, the clinicians decided to opt for rate control of the arrhythmia using a beta blocker. The risks and benefits of this treatment were explained. Metoprolol was chosen as an initial agent for rate control. The patient was admitted to hospital for assessment of her response to therapy and anti-coagulated on the basis of her $CHA_2DS_2VASc$ (3) and HAS-BLED (1) scores. Her response to metoprolol was good and she was changed over to regular bisoprolol 2.5 mg daily.

**Points to consider:**

- AF may present in general practice, acute medical wards or the emergency department.
- Haemodynamic stability of the patient must be assessed and rhythm versus rate control must be determined.
- The presence of mild COPD is not an absolute contraindication to the use of a beta-blocker, as this will not necessarily cause broncho-spasm; metoprolol was chosen as it has a short half-life.
- Digoxin was not considered suitable, as she was an active lady.
- Clinicians can use a combination of patient preference and validated tools such as HAS-BLED and $CHA_2DS_2VASc$ to determine the most appropriate management for thromboprophylaxis.

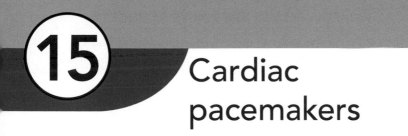

# Cardiac pacemakers

## 15.1 TYPES OF PACEMAKERS

### TRANSCUTANEOUS TEMPORARY PACING

- This can be carried out simply by applying pads in the anterior and posterior chest positions using automated external defibrillators.
- The rate and the lowest energy output to achieve capture must be set.
- It is uncomfortable for the patient who also experiences pectoral and skeletal muscle contraction, and therefore should only be used in the emergency setting.

### TRANSVENOUS TEMPORARY PACING

- A pacing wire is inserted aseptically via the venous system (e.g. femoral vein/jugular vein) into the right ventricle and attached to a pacemaker outside the body.

### TEMPORARY EPICARDIAL PACING

- This is the placement of pacing leads on the epicardium (outer surface) of the heart during open heart surgery.

### PERMANENT PACEMAKER

- Pacing leads are inserted into the heart chambers (right ventricle +/– right atrium) via a major venous branch under fluoroscopy guidance (usually left subclavian vein).
- The generator box is usually placed in a subcutaneous or submuscular pocket on the anterior chest wall below the clavicle under local anaesthetic.
- The leads are then inserted into the box and the pocket is surgically closed.

## 15.2 ADDITIONAL FEATURES OF A PERMANENT PACEMAKER

### DEFIBRILLATION

- An implantable cardiac defibrillator (ICD) may detect tachycardia and deliver a shock to restore sinus rhythm.
- ICDs can also function as a pacemaker.

## ANTI-TACHYCARDIA PACING (OVERDRIVE PACING)

- Modern ICDs are able to detect the difference between VF and VT.
- For VT, they may pace the heart at a faster rate than the arrhythmia to break the circuit before VT degenerates to VF.

## CARDIAC RESYNCHRONIZATION THERAPY

- Cardiac resynchronization therapy is useful in patients with severe heart failure with electrophysiological evidence of dyssynchrony caused by left bundle branch block.
- This conduction abnormality impairs efficient left ventricular contraction because the interventricular septum contracts out of synchrony with the free ventricular wall.
- A lead is introduced into the right ventricle via the venous system and another is passed through the coronary sinus into a cardiac vein, which thus allows the left ventricle to be paced directly.
- The ventricles are then paced individually but simultaneously to affect synchronous contraction of the septum with the free left ventricular wall.
- Strict criteria for this technique have been developed and are discussed on p. 74.

# 15.3 INTERNATIONAL CODING SYSTEM

| First letter | Chamber paced (V = ventricles, A = atria, D = dual) |
|---|---|
| Second letter | Chamber sensed (V = ventricles, A = atria, D = dual, O = none) |
| Third letter | Pacing response triggered from sensing activity (I = inhibited, T = triggered, D = dual, O = none) |
| Fourth letter | Programmable to respond to physiological changes |
| Fifth letter | Response if tachycardia is sensed (P = anti-tachycardia pacing, S = shock, D = dual, O = none) |

- Generally, patients who do not have coordinated atrial activity (atrial flutter or atrial fibrillation) receive a VVI pacemaker (pace ventricles, sense ventricles, pacing is inhibited if native activity is sensed).
- Other arrhythmias such as sick sinus syndrome where there is no degree of AV block will need an AAIR pacemaker (pace atria, sense atria, inhibit pacing if they sense activity and are rate-responsive).

- However, in most cases these patients and all those with dysfunction at and below the level of the AV node will receive a DDDR (pace both chambers, sense both, can both trigger and inhibit and are rate-responsive).
- Note that patients with sick sinus syndrome may later develop AV block.
- During surgery, electrocautery may be sensed by a pacemaker as an R wave and the pacemaker may therefore be inhibited – pacemakers may need to be switched to a VOO or DOO mode so they pace the chambers irrespective of what they sense for the duration of the procedure (this should be discussed with the surgeon to determine the type of diathermy being used and the location of use with respect to the heart).

## 15.4 EXAMPLES OF INDICATIONS

- Symptomatic sinus node dysfunction with significant pauses (≥3 seconds).
- Symptomatic high degree AV node dysfunction.
- Third-degree heart block irrespective of symptoms except in younger patients with a high nodal escape rhythm.
- Symptomatic bifascicular or trifascicular block with evidence of higher degree AV block.
- MI with **persistent** higher degree AV block.
- Cardiac conditions requiring medication therapy resulting in symptomatic bradycardia.
- Some forms of drug-resistant tachycardias.

### THE PACED ECG

- An atrial or ventricular upright pacing spike may be followed by a P or QRS wave.
- Ventricular pacing results in a wide QRS complex (see Figure 15.1).

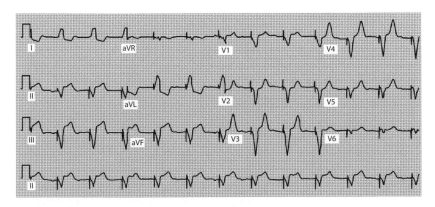

**Figure 15.1** Image of paced ECG.

Cardiology and the cardiovascular system

# 15.5 COMPLICATIONS

- *Insertion-related:*
  - Haematoma
  - Pneumothorax
  - Cardiac tamponade
  - Infection
  - Pocket erosion
- *Pacemaker syndrome:*
  - Is a result of AV dyssynchrony, or a lack of optimal timing between atrial and ventricular contraction leading to decreased cardiac output and resulting symptoms.
  - Usually occurs when there is ventricular pacing alone, in which case the native atria may even contract against a closed AV valve.
  - Dyssynchrony may even occur in the case of dual-chamber pacing.
- *Pacemaker-mediated tachycardia:*
  - Traditionally, this term referred to an artificial re-entrant loop tachycardia caused by a dual chamber pacemaker.
  - The pacemaker paces the atria and then the ventricles, but the ventricular activation then conducts retrogradely via the AV node to depolarize the atria again and a loop tachycardia results.
  - Management strategies include programming the pacemaker to avoid sensing retrogradely conducted P waves or switching the pacemaker to a single chamber one.

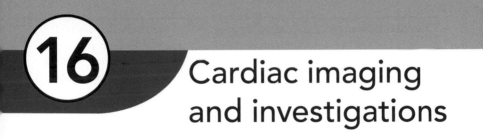

# Cardiac imaging and investigations

Heart imaging can offer both structural and functional information about the heart and its structures.

## 16.1 PLAIN CHEST RADIOGRAPH (CHEST X-RAY, CXR)

- An inexpensive test that is readily available and interpretable by most medical staff.
- It exposes the patient to a radiation dose equivalent to 10 days of background radiation.
- It is dependent on individual interpretation.
- The following features may be appreciated:

| Cardiac silhouette | A postero-anterior CXR gives a good impression of the overall size of the heart. Hypertrophy without ventricular enlargement rarely leads to radiologically evident enlargement. |
|---|---|
| Pericardial effusion | Pericardial effusion gives a classic image of a 'globular' heart. The edge of the heart is unusually crisp due to the fluid reducing movement artefact. See Figure 7.2 for an example. |
| Atrial dilatation | RA enlargement is classically due to right heart failure and tricuspid regurgitation. LA is the only chamber that may be accurately identified as a flattening and later bulging of the left heart border with elevation of the left main bronchus. The double-density sign occurs when there is the appearance of a double border on the right heart border resulting from the enlargement of the LA. |

*Continued*

| Vascular dilatation | An unfolded appearance of the thoracic aorta is common in the elderly due to dilatation and lengthening. A widened mediastinum may indicate aortic aneurysm or dissection. Pulmonary arteries may be dilated in pulmonary hypertension. |
| --- | --- |
| Intracardiac calcification | Calcification accompanies a number of disease processes. Pericardial calcification may accompany tuberculosis. Calcified valves may be apparent and may indicate damage. |
| Lung fields | Pulmonary congestion may be apparent due to pulmonary oedema. |

## MICRO-facts

The cardiac silhouette should not exceed 50% of the total lateral dimension of the chest on a posterior–anterior (PA) film. Silhouette size cannot be commented on in anterior–posterior (AP) films due to the potential for magnification.

# 16.2 ECHOCARDIOGRAPHY

- *Working principle:*
    - Echocardiography relies on ultrasound waves and their reflection off cardiac structures to create an image of the heart, which is received and interpreted by the operator in real time.

## TRANSTHORACIC ECHOCARDIOGRAPHY (TTE)

- The patient is usually rolled slightly to the left to bring the heart forward.
- The main views obtained in transthoracic echocardiography are (see Figure 16.1):
    - **Parasternal view:** the probe is placed in the vicinity of the second to fourth intercostal spaces at the left sternal edge to show the LA, LV, right outflow tract and aorta.
    - **Apical view:** the probe is placed at the fifth intercostal space in the midclavicular line to visualize the four-chamber view of the heart.
    - **Subcostal view:** the probe is placed just below the xiphisternum and visualizes a four-chamber view with an overlying liver.
    - **Suprasternal view:** the probe is placed over the suprasternal notch and shows the aortic arch.

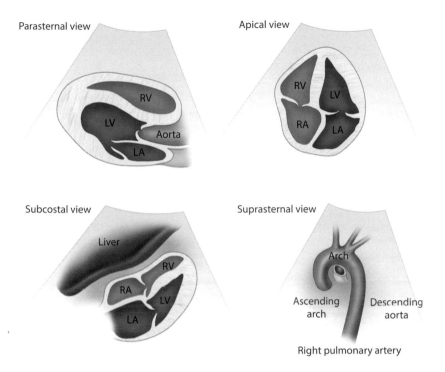

**Figure 16.1** Transthoracic echocardiogram views of the heart.

Doppler echocardiography

- Doppler can give information about blood flow within the heart and its vessels.
- The frequency of reflected ultrasound waves increases if red cells are moving towards the probe, allowing for the assessment of the direction of flow of blood.
- The change in frequency can be used to calculate the velocity of blood moving through cardiac valves.

---

## MICRO-facts

*Pulse wave Doppler* measures velocity at a pre-defined depth or specific point in the heart by pulsing short bursts of waves at this point.

- Good at measuring flow through the mitral valve and left ventricular outflow tract

*Continuous wave Doppler* measures velocity at all depths.

- It can calculate higher velocities and is useful in assessing stenotic valves.

*continued…*

---

Cardiology and the cardiovascular system

*continued...*

*Colour flow Doppler* imposes Doppler information on top of a 2D image of the heart.

- Velocities become colour-coded.
- Blood flow towards the probe is red.
- Blood flow away from the probe is blue.
- This is useful for identifying small high velocity jets such as in:
  - Aortic regurgitation
  - Mitral regurgitation
  - Ventricular septal defect

*Tissue Doppler* allows analysis of motion velocity of individual myocardial segments.

- May allow an estimation of LV systolic and diastolic dysfunction.
- Allows assessment of dyssynchrony in contraction to help evaluate if patients in heart failure would benefit from cardiac resynchronization therapy.

| USES FOR TRANSTHORACIC ECHOCARDIOGRAPHY | |
|---|---|
| **Evaluation of LV function** | Careful examination can allow an assessment of wall motion throughout the ventricle. Regional defects in wall motion are the hallmark of coronary artery disease. An estimate of which artery may be affected can be made dependent on which regions are affected. Signs of cardiomyopathies such as dilatation and hypertrophy are readily identified. |
| **Evaluation of RV abnormalities** | The dimensions and flow through the right ventricle RV may be recorded. The presence of pulmonary hypertension can be screened for by measuring the velocity of tricuspid regurgitation (pressure gradient = $4 V^2$). |
| **Assessment of heart valves** | Echocardiography is the gold standard test for assessing the function of the valves. It can screen for defects and quantify the severity of dysfunction, as well as help identify vegetations. |
| **Assessment of structural abnormalities** | Doppler echocardiography in particular can help to look for abnormal communications between the left and right sides of the heart. |

## TRANS-OESOPHAGEAL ECHOCARDIOGRAPHY (TOE)

- A trans-oesophageal echocardiogram involves passing a thin probe into the oesophagus to visualize the heart from the posterior aspect akin to endoscopy.
- It may require sedation to perform well.
- It provides clearer pictures due to the use of higher frequencies and the smaller tissue quantities that need to be penetrated.

| USES FOR TRANS-OESOPHAGEAL ECHOCARDIOGRAPHY | |
|---|---|
| **Assessment of valves** | TOE can aid diagnosis of infective endocarditis if vegetations are not seen on transthoracic echocardiogram but clinical suspicion remains high or the valves are prosthetic. It can aid preoperative assessment of the mitral valve. |
| **Assessment for cardio-embolic events** | TOE helps the search for an embolic source in an unexplained stroke in a young patient. It can visualize thrombi within the atria, atrial appendages and LV. |
| **Assessment of the aorta** | It can help in the assessment of acute dissection of the aorta. |
| **Assessment of structure** | TOE can assess the inter-atrial septum and look for a patent foramen ovale. It can delineate congenital heart disease and cardiac masses. |

## CONTRAST ECHOCARDIOGRAPHY

- Contrast echocardiography utilizes agitated saline or other contrast agents to aid visualization.
- Micro-bubbles in the contrast alter the appearance of the contrast as it passes through the heart from the venous circulation where it is injected.
- Micro-bubbles do not usually pass through the pulmonary system so their presence in the left side of the heart indicates the possibility of an intracardiac defect (e.g. atrial septal defect) that allows blood to shunt from right to left.
- Newer contrast agents that pass through the pulmonary system can help to define an LV thrombus.

## STRESS ECHOCARDIOGRAPHY

- Stress echocardiography is similar to perfusion imaging.
- Echocardiography assessment of both regional and global LV function is undertaken to look for evidence of coronary disease that affects ventricular function under imposed stress.

Cardiology and the cardiovascular system

- Each ventricle is divided into 16 segments which are graded individually.
- Segments are examined both at rest and under stress to identify wall motion abnormalities that develop with stress:
  - **Anterior** wall defects point towards disease in the left anterior descending artery.
  - **Lateral** wall defects point towards disease in the circumflex artery.
  - **Inferior** and **right ventricular** abnormalities point towards disease in the right coronary artery.
- Exercise or pharmacological agents are used to stress the heart.
- Pharmacological agents include dobutamine, a sympathomimetic drug.

# 16.3 CARDIAC CT

- Imaging options based on CT modality include plain CT, CT aortogram, CT pulmonary angiography, coronary CT angiography and coronary artery calcium scoring.
- In contrast to echocardiography, CT is unaffected by body habitus.

| USES FOR CARDIAC CT | |
|---|---|
| **Assessment for aortic disease** | CT with contrast is the imaging of choice for detecting aortic dissection. It can image the whole of the thoracic and abdominal aorta. It is superior to echocardiography, which may not image past the thoracic aorta, is invasive and may require sedation and an expert operator. |
| **Assessment for pericardial disease** | CT readily identifies calcification and allows the thickness of the pericardium to be assessed. Pericardial thickening and calcification is difficult to assess on echocardiography. |
| **Assessment for pulmonary embolism** | CT scanning with contrast (CT pulmonary angiography) is the gold standard for the diagnosis of both acute and chronic pulmonary embolism. These may result in pulmonary hypertension and right heart failure. |
| **Assessment for coronary artery disease** | This can be done either through the use of non-contrast CT coronary artery calcium scoring or CT coronary angiography. |

## CORONARY CT ANGIOGRAPHY

- Contrast is injected peripherally and CT images of the heart are captured, which may be reconstructed into a 3D image.

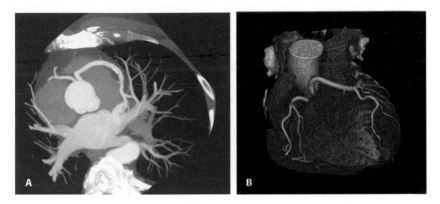

**Figure 16.2** Coronary CT angiography showing an anatomical anomaly where the left main stem arises from the anterior coronary sinus alone with the right coronary artery (A). A 3D reconstruction is also shown (B).

- 'Gating' of images with ECG allows minimization of cardiac movement artefact.
- A beta-blocker may be given to the patient to slow heart rate and allow better visualization.
- The radiation exposure of one scan is equivalent to 4 years of background radiation.
- Coronary CT angiography may be employed for the assessment of coronary artery disease, suspected coronary anomalies, restenosis in coronary stents or coronary artery bypass graft patency.
- It may also be used for coronary vein mapping for the purpose of planning the placement of a biventricular pacemaker (see Figure 16.2).

## CORONARY ARTERY CALCIUM SCORING

- Coronary artery calcium scoring by CT is increasingly recognized as a test for the investigation of low-risk chest pain (see Section 3.4).
- Intravenous contrast is not used.
- The radiation exposure of one scan is equivalent to 1 year of background radiation.
- It can show early coronary artery disease by looking for calcified atherosclerotic plaques in the arteries.
- It is a test that shows the presence of atherosclerotic disease but it is unable to comment on its physiological significance.

# 16.4 CARDIAC MRI

- Cardiac MRI use is limited by its availability, increased scan times, expense and need for specialist personnel.
- There is no exposure to ionizing radiation.

- Contraindications to use include implants such as pacemakers and defibrillators, although modern devices may be MRI compatible.
- Image quality is decreased by implants such as metallic valves and sternal wires even if it is deemed to be safe to perform MRI in patients with these after discussion with radiographers.
- MRI allows dynamic images of cardiac wall motion and blood flow.

| | |
|---|---|
| **Assessment for ventricular function and character** | Cardiac MRI can assess for ventricular volumes and function, including diastolic dysfunction. It is possible to assess for dilated cardiomyopathy, infiltrative cardiomyopathy such as amyloidosis, and ventricular hypertrophy. |
| **Assessment for cardiac structure** | Cardiac MRI can image congenital heart disease, valvular heart disease, aortic disease such as aneurysms, cardiac tumours and thrombi. |
| **Assessment for myocarditis and pericardial disease** | Cardiac MRI is the first-line imaging technique for the diagnosis of myocarditis. Features noted include hyperaemia, myocardial oedema and myocardial necrosis. The pericardium also shows up on MRI scanning although CT scanning may be better for demonstrating calcification. Cine views may be able to show the physiological effect of pericardial constrictive pathology on interventricular septal movement. |
| **Assessment for myocardial ischaemia** | Stress venticulography assesses for new regional wall motion abnormalities with cine views during periods of stress induced with agents such as dobutamine. Stress perfusion MRI can also be used to assess for myocardial ischaemia. Gadolinium contrast agent is injected intravenously and areas of myocardial ischaemia (produced by a pharmacological stressing agent such as adenosine) are detected on the imaging. |
| **Assessment for myocardial viability** | When assessed with gadolinium, the extent of hyperenhancement of damaged tissue may be able to differentiate between infarcted myocardium and myocardium that is viable but stunned. This is particularly important as revascularization techniques such as a coronary artery bypass graft have much better clinical outcomes in patients with viable myocardium, such as yielding an improved ejection fraction. |

*Continued*

| Diagnosis of myocardial infarction | Cardiac MRI in the emergency department has been used in the detection of acute coronary syndrome. Its application in this setting is restricted by the difficulty in the practical provision of the equipment and personnel. |
|---|---|

# 16.5 NUCLEAR IMAGING

- Myocardial perfusion imaging is the most widely used form of nuclear imaging in cardiology.

| Assessment for coronary artery disease | Myocardial perfusion imaging such as single photon emission computed tomography (SPECT) is able to identify areas of reversible ischaemia to aid the diagnosis of coronary artery disease and also to guide revascularization decisions in those with known ischaemic heart disease. |
|---|---|
| Diagnosis of myocardial infarction | Although often not a practical resource in this setting due to the limitations of scanning an acutely unwell patient, nuclear imaging is able to assess infarct size in acute myocardial infarction. |
| Assessment of left ventricular ejection fraction | Radionuclide ventriculography is capable of allowing assessment of left ventricular ejection fraction. |

## SINGLE PHOTON EMISSION COMPUTED TOMOGRAPHY (SPECT)

- SPECT is a functional imaging test used for the detection of reversible and non-reversible ischaemic heart disease.
- Myocardial perfusion scintigraphy was the original nuclear planar imaging technique but has been largely superseded by SPECT, which is based on the same principle and is able to obtain 3D images with a rotating camera.
- *Working principle:*
    - An isotope such as thallium$^{201}$ or technetium$^{99}$ is injected intravenously and taken up by the myocardium.
    - Levels of the isotope are highest in viable, well-perfused myocardium and can be visualized with gamma cameras that detect internal radiation.
    - Ischaemic or infarcted areas do not take up the isotope as effectively.

Cardiology and the cardiovascular system

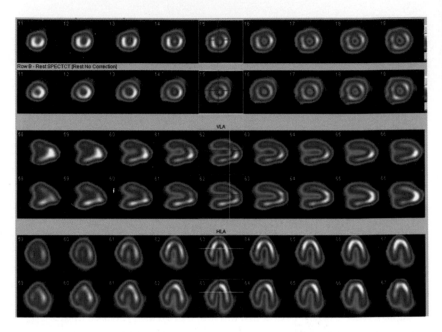

**Figure 16.3** SPECT images showing a stressed myocardium (upper panels) and myocardium at rest (lower panels). Note the difference in emission between the upper and lower panels, which indicates reversible myocardial ischaemia.

- The heart images can be compared at rest and during stress to reveal areas of reversible ischaemia or those with infarction (see Figure 16.3).
- Stress can be induced by either:
  - Exercise, or
  - Pharmacological agents:
    - Dobutamine
    - Arbutamine
    - Adenosine
    - Dipyridamole
- SPECT is less sensitive in the detection of multiple small vessel coronary artery disease.

## RADIONUCLIDE VENTRICULOGRAPHY

- This method of using scintigraphy consists of injecting technetium[99] intravenously and analysing its passage through the ventricles.
- The clearance of the radioactivity from the ventricles is related to the ejection fraction.

# 16.6 ANGIOGRAPHY

## RIGHT HEART CATHETERIZATION

- This invasive procedure used to be employed for the advancement of a Swan–Ganz balloon flotation catheter (first introduced in 1970) to aid in the assessment of cardiac haemodynamics particularly in patients with acute myocardial infarction.
- Due to its perceived ease of insertion and the information it yielded on cardiac haemodynamics, its use was widespread in the critically ill patient in the settings of sepsis, adult respiratory distress syndrome and post-surgery.
- Its use is much less widespread now.
- A catheter is inserted into either the femoral or basilic vein and advanced to the right atrium.
- Under fluoroscopy, it is advanced through the tricuspid valve up to the pulmonary artery.
- As an invasive procedure, there is a risk of serious complications including bleeding, infection, pneumothorax, haemothorax, coronary artery or pulmonary artery perforation or accidental insertion into the arterial circulation.
- Readings available include:
  - Pulmonary artery wedge pressure as an indirect assessment of left atrial pressures.
  - Pressures can be measured in each chamber of the right-sided chambers.
  - Estimates of cardiac output can be made.
  - Blood samples can be taken for oxygen saturation measurements.

| SOME CURRENT INDICATIONS |
| --- |
| For the diagnosis of pulmonary arterial hypertension |
| For use in patients with cardiogenic shock during supportive therapy |
| For cardiac transplantation work-up |
| For use in patients with suspected reversible systolic heart failure such as myocarditis |

## MICRO-facts

Oxygen saturations can be used to aid the diagnosis of the following:

- *Persistent ductus arteriosus* is indicated by higher saturations in the left pulmonary artery than the right ventricle.
- *Ventricular septal defects* are indicated by higher saturations in the pulmonary arteries and right ventricles than the right atrium.
- *Atrial septal defects* are indicated by higher saturations in the right atrium than in the vena cavae.

Cardiology and the cardiovascular system

## LEFT HEART CATHETERIZATION

- A catheter is placed in the arterial circulation through either the femoral or the radial arteries and advanced up to the aortic valve.
- The catheter may then be advanced past the valve into the ventricle or into the coronary ostia above the valve.

### Ventriculography and aortography

- Rapid injection of contrast media allows the visualization of the chambers and flow across the valves.
- Injection into the ventricle allows an estimation of LV function.
- Mitral regurgitation is apparent if contrast is seen in the LA after LV injection.
- Injection of media in the aorta above the valve will show aortic regurgitation if contrast flows back into the ventricle.

### Coronary angiography

- Coronary angiography is the most widely performed invasive cardiac investigation.
- It is used both to diagnose coronary disease and assess suitability for treatment either percutaneously or surgically.
- This is usually now carried out as a day case procedure for outpatient investigations.
- Over half of cases are now done via a radial approach instead of a femoral approach, leading to more rapid mobilization post-procedure and a decreased risk of bleeding.
- Contrast medium is injected and a variety of fluoroscopic images are taken to visualize distal run-off (see Figure 16.4).
- Coronary disease is seen as narrowing of the lumen with thinning of the contrast or as obstruction in the lumen with sudden cessation or tapering of contrast flow.
- Angiography may also be used to assess graft patency in patients who have undergone bypass surgery:
  - The technique is called selective angiography.
  - Specially shaped catheters are used to enter the left internal mammary artery and any vein grafts.

### MICRO-facts

Angiography risks:
- 1 in 2000 mortality
- 1 in 1000 risk of non-fatal stroke or myocardial infarction
- Local arterial complications are more common
  - Haematoma
  - False aneurysm
  - Dissections

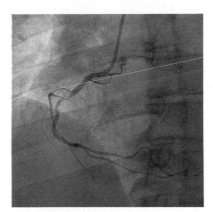

**Figure 16.4** Angiogram of the right coronary artery.

*Intravascular ultrasound*
- In some circumstances, an ultrasound probe mounted on a wire may be passed into the coronary arteries.
- This allows visualization of the arterial walls and can assess the composition of plaques.
- Evidence shows angiographically 'normal' arteries can in fact be significantly diseased.
- Pressure wires may be passed across a stenotic lesion to estimate its functional significance and assist with the decision to do angioplasty.

# 16.7 ELECTROPHYSIOLOGY

- Invasive electrophysiological testing involves positioning electrodes in locations around the heart, usually percutaneously via the venous system (may also use a trans-arterial route).
- Electrodes are positioned in the atria, ventricles and sites close to the conduction system.
- Allows identification of areas of increased or delayed conduction.

## PROVOCATION TESTING

- In some studies, stimuli are applied to the heart which may trigger arrhythmias.
- This is of use in:
  - Diagnosing arrhythmias by distinguishing the mechanisms of supraventricular tachycardias from one another.
  - Identification of specific trigger sites for ventricular arrhythmias or sites of bypass tracts such as in Wolff–Parkinson–White syndrome.

Cardiology and the cardiovascular system

- Testing the effectiveness of pharmacological therapies in preventing arrhythmias.
  - If a drug prevents an arrhythmia with provocation, it is likely to prevent the arrhythmia in future.
- Ablating the tissue responsible for provoking the arrhythmia can treat some arrhythmias, e.g. the bundle of Kent in Wolff–Parkinson–White syndrome.

---

**MICRO-case**

A 67-year-old man presented to his GP with increasing breathlessness over 6 months. He was a retired carpenter, moderately active and had a 30 pack-year smoking history (stopped 20 years ago). He had no significant past medical history. On examination, the cardiac apex was displaced, a pan-systolic murmur identified and bibasal crackles auscultated. The doctor requested a plain chest radiograph that revealed cardiomegaly and increased blood flow in upper lobe vessels. There were no further significant findings.

Venous blood samples were sent for FBC, U&E, TFT, LTF and serum natriuretic peptides (BNP/NTproBNP) in the absence of previous myocardial infarction. An ECG was also performed that revealed atrial fibrillation. The investigations strongly suggested a diagnosis of chronic heart failure and the GP organised an urgent transthoracic echocardiogram and cardiology referral. The echocardiogram showed severe mitral regurgitation.

The patient began medical treatment and was scheduled for valve replacement. The patient experienced a sudden worsening of his breathlessness and was admitted to hospital. A chest radiograph revealed cardiomegaly as previously noted, a pleural effusion, peri-hilar alveolar oedema and Kerley B lines. An urgent echocardiogram demonstrated chordae tendinae rupture. The patient was referred urgently to cardiothoracic surgeons.

**Points to consider:**

- Consider carefully the indications for requesting investigations such as radiographs and echocardiograms.
- Consider the use of tests in both urgent and non-urgent situations.

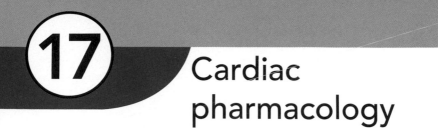

# Cardiac pharmacology

## 17.1 ANTI-ANGINAL

### PHYSIOLOGICAL BACKGROUND

- Angina is a mismatch between myocardial oxygen utilization and supply.
- Therapeutic targets include decreasing myocardial oxygen demand and increasing its supply.

| Factors influencing myocardial $O_2$ demand: <br> • Cardiac contractility (inotropy) <br> • Cardiac rate (chronotropy) <br> • Afterload and preload (affect ventricular work) | Therapeutic target: <br> • Decreasing inotropy <br> • Decreasing chronotropy <br> • Decreasing afterload and preload (vasodilatation) |
| --- | --- |
| Factors influencing myocardial $O_2$ supply: <br> • Coronary artery diameter (reduced in atheromatous disease and spasm) | Therapeutic target: <br> • Vasodilatation of coronary arteries |

- The following classes are anti-anginals (see Figure 17.1):
  - Nitrates
  - Calcium channel blockers
  - Beta-blockers
  - $K^+$ channel activators
  - Ivabradine
  - Ranolazine

### Nitrates
*Short-acting nitrates*
*Glyceryl trinitrate (GTN sublingual tablet/spray, IV infusion, transdermal patch)*

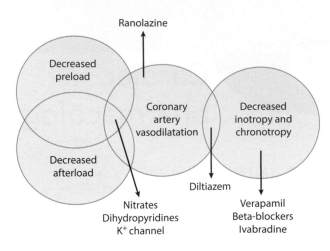

**Figure 17.1** Anginal medication.

## Long-acting nitrates
*Isosorbide mononitrate (ISMN), isosorbide dinitrate (ISDN) (sublingual tablet, oral)*

| Mode of action: | CVS therapeutic use: |
|---|---|
| • First-pass metabolism in the body produces nitrite ions that within vascular smooth muscle cells are converted to nitric oxide, a powerful vasodilator through its action on cyclic GMP. | • Angina |
| | • Pulmonary oedema in acute heart failure |
| | Non-CVS use: |
| • Decreases preload by venous pooling and increases myocardial $O_2$ supply by dilating coronary vessels. | • Anal fissure (GTN) |

Side effects:
- ▪ • Postural hypotension    → Caused by increased venous pooling of blood
- ▪ • Headaches, tachycardia, dizziness    → Effects of vasodilatation
- ▫ • Flushing    → Effects of vasodilatation
- ▪ • Angle-closure glaucoma    → Due to a rise in intraocular pressure

Beware:
- • Tolerance may develop with sustained use.
- • To be avoided in hypotensive patients.
- • Not to be used in combination with other potent vasodilators such as sildenafil.

## Calcium channel blockers

Differ in their selectivity for myocardial cells and vascular smooth muscle cells

| Vascular smooth muscle | | Myocardium and AV node |
|---|---|---|
| **Dihydropyridines**<br>Nifedipine, amlodipine | **Benzothiazepine**<br>Diltiazem | **Phenylalkylamine**<br>Verapamil |

| Mode of action: | CVS therapeutic use: |
|---|---|
| • Block the L (long) type calcium channels in heart muscle and vascular smooth muscle, reducing calcium influx and contractility.<br>• In the myocardium, this reduces cardiac inotropy and chronotropy.<br>• In the vessels, this causes vasodilatation, improving coronary flow and reducing afterload and preload. | • Angina<br>Dihydropyridines:<br>• Hypertension<br>• Coronary vasospasm<br>• Cerebral vasospasm<br>• Raynaud's syndrome<br>Verapamil, diltiazem<br>• Supraventricular tachycardia (SVT) |

Side effects:

Dihydropyridines

- Nausea
- Peripheral oedema, flushing → Due to increased venous pooling of blood
- Palpitations → Manifestation of reflex sympathetic activation and tachycardia mediated by the baroreceptors
- Postural hypotension → Effect of vasodilatation
- Angioedema → Due to increased venous pooling of blood

Verapamil, diltiazem

- Constipation → Effect on gut muscle, decreased contraction
- Bradycardia, heart block → Excessive negative chronotropic effect
- Rash

Beware:
- Do not prescribe verapamil/diltiazem with beta-blockers as this may cause significant bradycardia (occasionally heart block, especially in the elderly).
- Avoid verapamil/diltiazem in heart failure as they are negatively inotropic.
- Use of dihydropyridines in severe aortic stenosis may reduce cardiac output due to vasodilatation.

Cardiology and the cardiovascular system

## Potassium channel activators
*Nicorandil*

| Mode of action: | CVS therapeutic use: |
|---|---|
| • K⁺ channels are located on vascular smooth muscle cells and allow K⁺ to exit the cell – this hyperpolarizes the membrane and results in vasodilatation. | • Angina |

Side effects:
■ • Headache, flushing → Effect of vasodilatation
■ • Nausea and vomiting
■ • GI ulceration (oral, anal) → Unknown mechanism

Beware:
• Avoid in hypotensive patients.

## Beta-blockers
*Atenolol, metoprolol, carvedilol, bisoprolol*

> **MICRO-print**
> Different adrenergic receptors, location and effect of stimulation
>
> | $\alpha_1$ Receptor | Smooth muscle | Contraction (vascular) |
> |---|---|---|
> | $\alpha_2$ Receptor | Smooth muscle, CNS | Stops neurotransmitter release |
> | $\beta_1$ Receptor | Myocardium | ↑Chronotropy and inotropy |
> | $\beta_2$ Receptor | Smooth muscle | Relaxation (airway and vascular) |
> | $\beta_3$ Receptor | Fat | Lipolysis |

> **MICRO-facts**
> Beta-blockers have different side-effect profiles depending on properties:
> • May have intrinsic sympathomimetic activity resulting in less side effects of cold extremity (celiprolol)
> • ↑Water-solubility will ↓blood–brain barrier crossing (atenolol).
> • ↑Cardioselectivity (less $\beta_2$ effect) will reduce bronchospasm (atenolol, bisoprolol, carvedilol; propranolol is very non-selective).

| Mode of action: | CVS therapeutic use: |
|---|---|
| • Inhibiting the stimulation of the $\beta_1$ receptors will decrease cardiac inotropy and chronotropy. | • Angina<br>• Post-MI<br>• Arrhythmias<br>• Heart failure<br>• Hypertension (no longer first-line)<br>Non-CVS uses:<br>• Thyrotoxicosis |

Side effects:

■ • Bronchospasm → Blocks $\beta_2$ receptors in airway smooth muscle

■ • Bad dreams and insomnia → Crosses blood–brain barrier

■ • Cold extremities → Blocks $\beta_2$ receptors in peripheral vasculature

■ • Bradycardia, heart block → Excessive blockage of $\beta_1$ receptors

■ • Decreased glucose tolerance → Effect possibly mediated by $\beta_3$ receptors

■ • Hypotension, erectile dysfunction → Blocks $\alpha$ receptors affecting blood pressure

■ • Psoriatiform rash

Beware:
- Avoid in asthma, heart block, bradycardia, unstable heart failure and critical limb ischaemia.
- Given in conjunction with thiazide diuretics may lead to glucose intolerance (controversial).
- Avoid giving with rate-limiting calcium channel blockers.

## Ivabradine

| Mode of action: | CVS therapeutic use: |
|---|---|
| • Blocks the $I_f$ 'funny' ion current in the sinoatrial node, decreasing pacemaker rate. | • Angina where beta-blockers are contraindicated<br>• Heart failure where beta-blockers are contraindicated |

Side effects:

■ • Bradycardia, first-degree heart block → Excessive block of the sinoatrial node

■ • Blurred vision

Beware:
- Avoid in heart block, sick sinus syndrome, bradycardia.

Ranolazine

| Mode of action: | CVS therapeutic use: |
|---|---|
| • Blocks late inward sodium currents in myocytes, reducing intracellular sodium and calcium that normally inhibit myocyte relaxation in ischaemia – relaxation of cardiac muscle lowers diastolic ventricular pressures and therefore allows better myocardial perfusion by alleviating compression of the myocardial blood supply. | • Stable angina |

Side effects:
- • Constipation, nausea, vomiting
- • Dizziness
- • Asthenia
- • Prolonged QT interval          → Prolongation of action potential

# 17.2 ANTI-HYPERTENSIVES

## PHYSIOLOGICAL BACKGROUND

- Maintenance of BP is essential to ensure provision of organ perfusion.
- The BP is controlled by arterial baroreceptors.
- BP is dependent on the pump (heart rate and contractility) and vasculature (preload, afterload and systemic vascular resistance).
- BP is controlled by both neurological and humeral mechanisms:
  - These are the factors upon which anti-hypertensive medications act.
- Drugs with anti-hypertensive properties include (see Figure 17.2):
  - Diuretics
  - ACEi and ARB
  - Calcium channel blockers (dihydropyridines, see p. 211)
  - Beta-blockers (see p. 212)
  - $\alpha_1$ Blockers
  - $\alpha_2$ Agonists
  - Minoxidil
  - Hydralazine
  - Nitroprusside

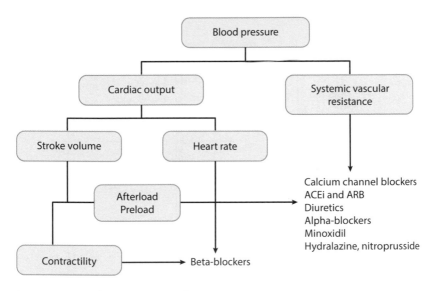

Figure 17.2 Anti-hypertensive medication.

## MICRO-facts

Generic rule for diuretics:

- Loss of sodium = Loss of water

Diuretics

- 100% of sodium is freely filtered from the glomerulus into the renal tubule in the nephron:
    - 65% is reabsorbed in the proximal convoluted tubule.
    - 25% is reabsorbed in the ascending loop of Henle.
    - 8% is reabsorbed at the distal convoluted tubule.
    - 2% is absorbed in the collecting duct.
    - <1% is excreted in normal health.
- Diuretics induce water loss (diuresis) by enhancing sodium excretion (natriuresis) (see Figure 17.3).
- Loop diuretics, thiazide diuretics and potassium-sparing diuretics are used in cardiology.

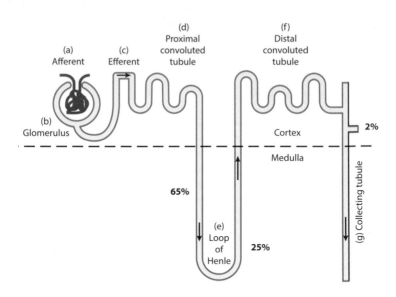

**Figure 17.3** Note the sections of the nephron and the percentage of total sodium reabsorbed in each nephron section. The loop diuretics act on the loop of Henle (e). Thiazide diuretics work on the distal convoluted tubule (f). Potassium-sparing diuretics act on the collecting tubules (g).

## Loop diuretics
*Furosemide, bumetanide*

| Mode of action: | CVS therapeutic use: |
|---|---|
| • Luminal membrane, ascending loop of Henle: NKCC2 ($Na^+/K^+/2Cl^-$) co-transporter channel is blocked, decreasing NaCl reabsorption. The medulla fails to concentrate enough to stimulate water reabsorption from the tubule.<br>• Induce venodilatation (increased prostaglandin production) systemically reducing preload and locally improving renal blood flow. | • Oedema in heart failure<br>• Hypertension<br>Non-CVS use:<br>• Oedema in liver cirrhosis, nephrotic syndrome<br>• Cerebral oedema<br>• Hypercalcaemia |

Side effects:
- ■ • Hyponatraemia and hypovolaemia → Powerful natriuresis and excess diuresis
- ■ • Hypokalaemia → Changes ionic gradients necessary to allow cation reabsorption
- ■ • Hypocalcaemia, hypomagnesaemia
- ■ • Reversible hearing loss (ototoxic) → Alters the ion gradient in endolymph
- ■ • Intrahepatic cholestasis

Beware:
- Hypokalaemia may precipitate cardiac arrhythmias and digoxin toxicity.
- Aminoglycosides are also ototoxic and may compound the ototoxic effect of loop diuretics.
- Caution in those with severe renal impairment.

## Thiazide and thiazide-like diuretics
### Indapamide, bendroflumethiazide, chlorthalidone

| Mode of action: | CVS therapeutic use: |
|---|---|
| • Luminal membrane, distal convoluted tubule NCC ($Na^+/Cl^-$) co-transporter channel is blocked, decreasing NaCl reabsorption.<br>• Arterial vasodilatation possibly by $K^+$ channel activation decreasing blood pressure. | • Hypertension<br>• Oedema in heart failure<br>Non-CVS use:<br>• Diabetes insipidus |

Side effects:
- Hyponatraemia            → Natriuresis
- Hypokalaemia             → Increases excretion of $K^+$
- Hypercalcaemia           → Low excretion, linked $Na^+$ and $Ca^{2+}$ reabsorption

- Precipitates gout        → Decreases uric acid excretion
- Impaired glucose tolerance → Possibly decreases insulin release
- Dyslipidaemia            → Increases triglycerides

Beware:
- Hypokalaemia may precipitate cardiac arrhythmias and digoxin toxicity.
- Thiazides given with beta-blockers increase the risk of precipitating diabetes (controversial).

---

**MICRO-print**

In both loop and thiazide diuretics, decreased $Na^+$ reabsorption and diuresis activates the renin–angiotensin system, increasing aldosterone production and action. This results in more $K^+$ and $H^+$ secretion in the distal convoluted tubule and collecting duct, resulting in side effects: *hypokalaemic metabolic alkalosis*.

---

# MICRO-facts

Chlorthalidone is a thiazide-related drug with a longer duration of action and more gentle effect on micturition frequency. Indapamide is a stronger vasodilator with a lesser effect on glucose tolerance.

## Potassium-sparing diuretics
*Spironolactone, eplerenone, amiloride*

| Mode of action: | CVS therapeutic use: |
|---|---|
| *ENaC blockers (amiloride)*<br>• Luminal membrane distal convoluted tubule and collecting duct ENaC channel (epithelial Na$^+$ channel) is blocked, decreasing Na$^+$ reabsorption.<br>*Aldosterone antagonists (spironolactone, eplerenone)*<br>• Aldosterone-antagonist decreasing expression of ENaC channel | • Hypertension<br>• Oedema in heart failure<br>• Chronic heart failure (spironolactone/ eplerenone)<br>Non-CVS use:<br>• Non-cardiac oedema, e.g. liver failure |

Side effects:
- ■ • Gastrointestinal disturbance
- ■ • Hyponatraemia     → Natriuresis
- ■ • Hyperkalaemia     → Sodium excess in tubule makes luminal potential less negative, decreasing K$^+$ secretion

Spironolactone only
- ■ • Hypertrichosis    → Reduces aldosterone anti-androgenic activity
- ■ • Gynaecomastia

Beware:
- • Giving potassium-sparing diuretics with ACE inhibitors increases risk of hyperkalaemia.

## Drugs acting on the renin–angiotensin–aldosterone axis
- Cells in the macula densa (specialized part of the distal convoluted tubule) detect the NaCl concentration in the filtrate.
- A low concentration stimulates renin release from the adjacent juxta-glomerular cells in the afferent arteriole.
- Renin cleaves angiotensinogen (produced by the liver and present in the blood) to angiotensin I, which is transformed into angiotensin II by angiotensin-converting enzymes (ACE) in the lungs.
- Effect of angiotensin II:
  - Systemic vasoconstriction
  - Constriction of the efferent arteriole raising glomerular pressure
  - Release of anti-diuretic hormone, allowing water retention
  - Stimulating the release of aldosterone, increasing sodium and water retention

*ACEi and ARBs*

*Ramipril, lisinopril, captopril, enalapril (ACEi), candesartan, losartan, irbesartan (ARB)*

| Mode of action: | CVS therapeutic use: |
|---|---|
| *ACE inhibitors* <br> • Antagonize ACE, reducing angiotensin II and aldosterone, inducing vasodilatation, inducing natriuresis and decreasing sympathetic activity. <br> *Angiotensin II receptor blockers (ARB)* <br> • Angiotensin II receptor antagonism | • Hypertension <br> • Congestive heart failure <br> • Post-MI (reduce deleterious remodelling) <br> Non-CVS use: <br> • Diabetic nephropathy |

Side effects:

- ■ • First-dose hypotension, headache, dizziness → Excess blocking of angiotensin II production
- ■ • Hyperkalaemia → Blockage of aldosterone production and decrease in K$^+$ secretion
- ■ • Teratogenic

ACEi only

- ■ • Dry cough → Increased bradykinins locally in lung tissue that are usually degraded by ACE
- ■ • Angioedema → More common in Afro-Caribbean patients

Beware:
- • Giving ACEi and ARB with potassium-sparing diuretics increases hyperkalaemia.
- • In bilateral renal artery stenosis can cause renal failure (removes efferent arteriole vasoconstriction by angiotensin II that is necessary to maintain glomerular pressure).
- • Do not use in pregnancy.
- • Less effective in the Afro-Caribbean population.

*Renin inhibitors*

*Aliskiren*

| Mode of action: | CVS therapeutic use: |
|---|---|
| • Inhibits the action of renin, stopping the conversion of angiotensinogen to angiotensin I | • Hypertension |

Side effects:
- ■ • Diarrhoea, rash
- • Rash
- ■ • Hyperkalaemia

Beware:
- • Like in ACEi and ARB, do not give to patients with renal artery stenosis and renal failure.

Cardiology and the cardiovascular system

## MICRO-facts

Check the following before starting someone on an ACEi, ARB or renin inhibitor:

- Serum creatinine good renal function
- Potassium U&E
- Exclude renal artery stenosis (auscultation)

### Drugs acting on alpha adrenergic receptors

#### $\alpha^1$ Blockers

*Doxazosin, prazosin*

| Mode of action: | CVS therapeutic use: |
|---|---|
| • Blocks the $\alpha$ receptors on vascular smooth muscle cells, resulting in vasodilatation | • Hypertension<br>Non-CVS use:<br>• Benign prostatic hypertrophy |

Side effects:

- First dose hypotension $\rightarrow$ Excess blocking of $\alpha$ receptors
- Oedema
- Palpitations
- Impotence $\rightarrow$ Excess blocking of $\alpha$ receptors

#### $\alpha^2$ Agonists/centrally acting anti-hypertensives

*Methyldopa, clonidine*

| Mode of action: | CVS therapeutic use: |
|---|---|
| • Stimulates presynaptic $\alpha_2$ receptors in the medulla, decreasing sympathetic output and resulting in reduced heart rate and vasodilatation | • Hypertension |

Side effects:

- Dry mouth, sedation $\rightarrow$ Low sympathetic output
- Bradycardia, postural hypotension $\rightarrow$ Effect of excessive vasodilatation
- Exacerbation of angina

Methyldopa

- Erectile dysfunction, galactorrhoea $\rightarrow$ Lowers dopamine production, allowing prolactin production

Beware:

- Stopping clonidine abruptly may precipitate a hypertensive crisis.
- Do not give methyldopa in active liver disease, depression or phaechromocytoma.

## Minoxidil

| Mode of action: | CVS therapeutic use: |
|---|---|
| • Activates ATP-sensitive K$^+$ channels, hyperpolarizing the vascular smooth muscle cell membranes and causing vasodilatation | • Hypertension |

Side effects:

■ • Fluid retention → Effect of vasodilatation in the peripheries

■ • Tachycardia → Reflex response to vasodilatation mediated by the baroreceptors

■ • Hypertrichosis → Unknown mechanism

Beware:

• Should be prescribed with a beta-blocker and diuretic to avoid tachycardia and fluid retention

## Hydralazine

| Mode of action: | CVS therapeutic use: |
|---|---|
| • Decreases release of Ca$^{2+}$ in vascular smooth muscle cell resulting in vasodilatation | • Severe hypertension<br>• Pregnancy hypertension<br>• Heart failure |

Side effects:

■ • Tachycardia, palpitations → Reflex response to vasodilatation mediated by baroreceptors

■ • Fluid retention → Effect of vasodilatation in the peripheries

■ • Rash

Beware:

• Drug-induced lupus erythematosus

## MICRO-facts

Note that nitrates act mainly on veins, versus hydralazine that acts mainly on arterioles

## Sodium nitroprusside

| Mode of action: | CVS therapeutic use: |
|---|---|
| • Given as an infusion, breaks down to NO in vascular smooth muscle resulting in vasodilatation. | • Severe hypertension<br>• Acute heart failure |

Side effects:

- ■ Headache, hypotension, dizziness  →  Effect of vasodilatation
- ■ Abdominal pain  →  Effect of rapid reduction in blood pressure
- ■ Palpitations

Beware:

- Do not give to patients with active liver disease or vitamin $B_{12}$ deficiency.
- In patients with Leber's optic neuropathy, use will aggravate optic ischaemia.

# 17.3 ANTI-ARRHYTHMICS

## PHYSIOLOGICAL BACKGROUND

- The Singh–Vaughan Williams classification is traditionally used to classify anti-arrhythmic drugs by mechanism of action.
- The different drugs act on the action potential in myocytes and pacemaker myocytes (see Figure 17.4):

| Class I | Block $Na^+$ channels | Ia: quinidine, procainamide<br>Ib: lignocaine<br>Ic: flecainide |
|---|---|---|
| Class II | Block $\beta_1$ receptors | Atenolol, metoprolol |
| Class III | Block $K^+$ channels | Amiodarone, sotalol |
| Class IV | Block $Ca^{2+}$ channels | Verapamil, diltiazem |
| Class V | Other mechanisms | Amiodarone, digoxin, atropine |

**MICRO-print**
Although the SVW classification is useful, some drugs act through more than one mechanism. It may be useful to classify by condition treated (from the British National Formulary):

- SVT: adenosine (class V), digoxin (class V), verapamil (class IV)
- SVT and VT: amiodarone (class III), beta-blockers (class II), classes Ia and Ic
- VT: class Ib and amiodarone
- Bradycardia: atropine

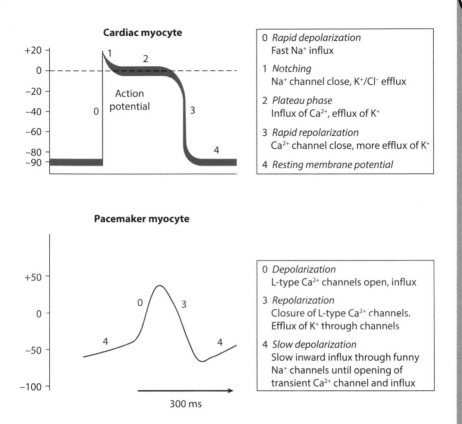

**Figure 17.4** Physiology of cardiac depolarization.

## Sodium channel blockers (class I)
### Class Ia – prolong action potential
*Quinidine, procainamide, disopyramide*

| Mode of action: | CVS therapeutic use: |
|---|---|
| • Block already open Na⁺ channels, slowing phase 0 and phase 4 in myocytes<br> • Widening the action potential<br>• ↓Inotropy<br>• ↓Atrial, AV node, His-Purkinje conduction<br>• ↑Refractory period (stopping re-entry tachycardias by making tissue less receptive) | • SVT, VT<br>Non-CVS therapeutic use<br>• Malaria (quinidine) |

Cardiology and the cardiovascular system

Side effects:

Quinidine

■ • Haemolytic anaemia, hepatitis,    → Immunological reaction
thrombocytopenia

Disopyramide

■ • Hypotension    → Peripheral $\alpha_1$ blockade

■ • Dry mouth, urine retention,    → Due to anti-cholinergic effects
constipation

Procainamide

■ • Drug-induced lupus erythematosus

■ • Agranulocytosis

Beware:
• Possible ECG changes: long PR and long QRS (avoid in AV block, sinoatrial disease).
• Prolonged QT interval (can precipitate torsades de pointes).
• Conchinism: effects of quinidine intoxication including tinnitus, delirium, visual disturbance.
• Do not give disopyramide to patients with glaucoma or benign prostatic hyperplasia (due to anti-cholinergic side effects), and heart failure or hypotension (negative inotropic).

### Class Ib – narrow action potential
*Lignocaine, phenytoin*

| Mode of action: | CVS therapeutic use: |
|---|---|
| • Block Na⁺ channels that are not yet open, slowing phase 0 in myocytes<br>  • Narrow the action potential<br>• ↑Refractory period<br>• No effect on AV node – no use in SVT | • Post-MI, VT<br>Non-CVS therapeutic use:<br>• Local anaesthetic (lignocaine)<br>• Epilepsy (phenytoin) |

Side effects:

Lignocaine

■ • Dizziness, paresthesia

■ • Nausea, vomiting

■ • Hypotension, bradycardia

■ • Anaphylaxis

Phenytoin

| | | | |
|---|---|---|---|
| ■ | • Tremor, nystagmus, sedation, ataxia | → | Effects are dose-related |
| ■ | • Gingival hypertrophy | → | Caused by folate deficiency due to enzyme inhibition |
| ■ | • Peripheral neuropathy | → | Caused by folate deficiency |
| ■ | • Hepatotoxicity | | |

Beware:
- ECG changes are possible – decreased corrected QT interval.
- Do not use in sinoatrial node disease and heart block.
- Lignocaine toxicity: paraesthesia, confusion, seizures.
- Need to reduce lignocaine dose in patients with chronic cardiac failure and liver failure.

*Class Ic – no effect on action potential duration*

*Flecainide*

| Mode of action: | CVS therapeutic use: |
|---|---|
| • Block $Na^+$ channels<br>No effect on the action potential duration<br>• ↓Inotropy<br>• ↓AV conduction<br>• No effect on refractory period | • SVT, VT |

Side effects:

| | | | |
|---|---|---|---|
| ■ | • Dizziness | | |
| ■ | • Visual disturbance | → | Unknown mechanism |

Beware:
- ECG changes are possible: prolonged PR, QRS and corrected QT.
- Do not use in patients with structural heart disease – precipitates ventricular arrhythmias.
- Do not use in patients with sinoatrial node disease and heart block.

## Potassium channel blockers (class III)

*Amiodarone, sotalol*

| Mode of action: | CVS therapeutic use: |
|---|---|
| • Block $K^+$ channels, slowing phase 0 and 3 in the myocytes<br> • Prolongs action potential<br>• ↓Refractory period<br>• Sotalol has beta-blocking effects | • SVT, VT |

Side effects:

Amiodarone

- Thyroid dysfunction → Drug contains iodine, stops conversion of T4 to T3

- Acute liver damage → Accumulation in liver
- Photosensitivity (slate-colour skin) → Accumulation in skin
- Pulmonary fibrosis → Amiodarone–phospholipid complexes that are engulfed by macrophages may characterize an interstitial pneumonitis

- Deposits in cornea and the eye that do not affect vision
- Peripheral neuropathy
- Optic neuritis (controversial)

Beware:
- Prolonged corrected QT (precipitates torsades de pointes).
- Do not use in patients with sinoatrial node disease and heart block.
- Sotalol has beta-blocking side effects and its class III effect is only significant at high doses.

## Adenosine (purine agonist)

| Mode of action: | CVS therapeutic use: |
|---|---|
| • Stimulates $A_1$ adenosine receptors<br>• Opens $K^+$ channels (hyperpolarizing cell) and inhibits $Ca^{2+}$ channels, slowing conduction through the AV node | • SVT |

Side effects:
- Dyspnoea, bronchospasm → Due to vagal effects
- Transient facial flushing, sweating → Effect of anti-adrenergic vasodilatation (short-lived)
- Metallic taste in mouth

Beware:
- ECG changes: increased PR interval (slow AV conduction).
- Do not use in patients with asthma, second- and third-degree heart block, sick sinus syndrome.

Digoxin (cardiac glycoside)

| Mode of action: | CVS therapeutic use: |
|---|---|
| • Inhibits Na$^+$/K$^+$ ATPase pump, increasing cellular Na$^+$ concentration and decreasing Ca$^{2+}$ excretion mediated by the Ca$^{2+}$/Na$^+$ pump – increased cellular Ca$^{2+}$ causes positive inotropy<br>  • Lengthens phases 0 and 4 of action potential in the myocyte<br>• Increase vagal stimulation of AV node, thereby slowing conduction and heart rate | • SVT<br>• Heart failure |

Side effects:

■ • Nausea, vomiting, diarrhoea (over dosage) → Due to increased vagal effects

 • Depression

Beware:

• ECG changes: increased PR interval (slow AV conduction).
• Hypokalacmia potentiates digoxin as K$^+$ is a competitor at the Na$^+$/K$^+$ ATPase pump, beware use with hypokalaemia-inducing loop and thiazide diuretics.
• Do not use in patients with Wolff–Parkinson–White syndrome or heart block.

---

**MICRO-facts**

Digoxin has a narrow therapeutic range. Digoxin toxicity results in visual blurring, yellow vision (xanthopsia), nausea and vomiting, abdominal pain, headaches and delirium. ECG characteristic change is upsloping ST segment depression (reverse tick sign). It may result in arrhythmias. Treat with digoxin-specific antibody fragments (Digibind®).

---

Atropine

| Mode of action: | CVS therapeutic use: |
|---|---|
| • Competitive antagonist of the muscarinic acetylcholine receptors that slows down pacemaker activity at the sino-atrial node | • Bradycardia<br>Non-CVS use:<br>• Reversing neuromuscular block<br>• Organophosphate toxicity<br>• Iritis |

Cardiology and the cardiovascular system

Side effects:

■ • Dry mouth, double-vision, urinary retention, constipation, bradycardia → Due to anti-cholinergic side effects

■ • Angle-closure glaucoma → Raised intraocular pressure due to anti-cholinergic mechanism

Beware:
- Link the anti-cholinergic side effects to the contraindications: do not use in paralytic ileus (constipation), benign prostatic hyperplasia (urinary retention), myasthenia gravis and glaucoma (raised intraocular pressure).

# 17.4 ANTI-COAGULANTS AND THROMBOLYTIC AGENTS

## PHYSIOLOGICAL BACKGROUND

- The coagulation cascade has three components: intrinsic, extrinsic and common pathway (see Figure 17.5).
- **In-green** factors produced by the liver and dependent on vitamin K.
- **In-red** factors that can be acted on to inhibit coagulation.
- Plasminogen produced by the liver can be converted to plasmin by tissue plasminogen activator (tPA) found in endothelial cells lining blood vessels.
- Plasmin is an enzyme that cleaves fibrin clots.

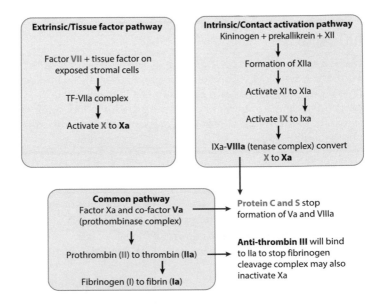

Figure 17.5 Clotting cascade.

## Warfarin

| Mode of action: | CVS therapeutic use: |
|---|---|
| • Vitamin K antagonist.<br>• Vitamin K works as a co-factor in the production of factors II (prothrombin), VII, IX and X and proteins C and S. | • DVT, PE treatment and prophylaxis<br>• Prosthetic heart valve<br>• Atrial fibrillation |

Side effects:

- Haemorrhage → Excess anti-coagulation
- Skin necrosis → Paradoxical blood clotting reduces blood supply to the skin
- Purple toes → Unclear mechanism

Beware:

- Do not use in patients with active haemorrhage, peptic ulcers and severe hypertension.
- Teratogenic.
- To reverse warfarin overdose use vitamin K (phytomenadione) and for quicker onset of action use prothrombin complex concentrate (factors II, VII, IX, X and proteins C and S) or fresh frozen plasma.

## Unfractionated heparin (UFH) and low-molecular-weight heparins (LMWHs)

*Enoxaparin, dalteparin (LMWHs)*

| Mode of action: | CVS therapeutic use: |
|---|---|
| • Speeds up the formation of anti-thrombin III and thrombin (IIa), inactivating thrombin.<br>• Heparin–antithrombin III complexes inhibit factor Xa (only action of LMWH).<br>• LMWHs have a longer half-life. | • DVT, PE<br>• Unstable angina, NSTEMI<br>• Surgical prophylaxis<br>• Acute peripheral artery occlusion |

Side effects:

- Haemorrhage → Excess anti-coagulation
- HITT (heparin-induced thrombocytopenia and thrombosis) → Formation of antibodies activating platelets
- Injection site reaction and skin necrosis → From subcutaneous administration

Beware:
- Do not give in haemophilia, thrombocytopenia and other haemorrhagic disorders.
- Do not give in active internal bleeding, severe hypertension and peptic ulcer disease.
- Do not allow a patient to have spinal or epidural anaesthesia on heparin due to risk of haematoma and spinal cord compression.

---

**MICRO-facts**

**PT (prothrombin time)**

Measures the activity of the extrinsic pathway, affected by vitamin K-dependent factors (II, VII, IX, X)

**INR (international normalized ratio) for warfarin**

INR is a standardized method of expressing PT compared to a standard and is used to monitor warfarin effect (e.g. an INR of 2.0 means the PT is twice as long compared with a control)

**APTT (activated partial thromboplastin time) for heparin**

Measures the activity of the intrinsic and common pathways

---

Novel anti-coagulants

- Their oral formulations and quick onset of action make it unnecessary to monitor markers of anti-coagulation (unlike routine monitoring of international normalized ratios in warfarin use).
- Unlike vitamin K use in warfarin overdose, there is no known therapeutic agent that will reverse the effect of these agents in situations of overdose or uncontrolled bleeding, but several promising agents are currently in research and trial.
- They cost more than warfarin.

*Factor X inhibitor*

*Dabigatran*

| Mode of action: | CVS therapeutic use: |
|---|---|
| • Direct inhibitor of factor X (thrombin) in the platelet cascade | • Stroke and systemic emboli prevention in non-valvular atrial fibrillation |

Side effects:
- Nausea
- Abdominal pain, dyspepsia, diarrhoea
- Epistaxis, other bleeding, anaemia → Excess anti-coagulation
- Possible increased risk of myocardial infarction → Unknown mechanism

Beware:
- Do not give to patients with compromised haemostasis.
- Not for patients with severe hepatic or renal dysfunction.
- Not to be used concomitantly with ketoconazole, ciclosporin, itraconazole or tacrolimus.

---

**MICRO-reference**

Evidence for the non-inferiority of dabigatran compared to warfarin for stroke and systemic emboli prevention in patients with non-valvular atrial fibrillation comes from the RE-LY trial. See: Connolly SJ, Ezekowitz MD, Yusuf S, et al. Dabigatran versus warfarin in patients with atrial fibrillation. *The New England Journal of Medicine* 2009; 361: 1139–1151.

---

**MICRO-facts**

NICE guidelines recommend the use of dabigatran in patients where warfarin use is not recommended and patients have one of the following risk factors:

- Previous stroke, transient ischaemic attack or systemic embolism
- Left ventricular ejection fraction below 40%
- Symptomatic heart failure of New York Heart Association (NYHA) class 2 or above
- Age 75 years or above
- Age 65 years or over with one of the following: diabetes mellitus, coronary artery disease or hypertension

National Institute for Health and Care Excellence. Atrial fibrillation: the management of atrial fibrillation. NICE guidelines [CG180]. London: National Institute for Health and Care Excellence, 2014.

---

*Factor Xa inhibitors*

*Rivaroxaban, apixaban*

| Mode of action: | CVS therapeutic use: |
|---|---|
| • Direct inhibitor of factor Xa (prothrombin) | • Stroke and systemic emboli prevention in non-valvular atrial fibrillation |

Side effects:
- Nausea
- Bleeding, anaemia → Excess anti-coagulation
- Transaminitis (rivaroxaban)

Beware:
- Do not give to patients with compromised haemostasis.
- Not for patients with severe hepatic or renal dysfunction.

---

**MICRO-references**

Evidence for the non-inferiority of rivaroxaban compared to warfarin for stroke and systemic embolism prevention in patients with non-valvular atrial fibrillation comes from the ROCKET-AF trial. See: Patel MR, Mahaffey KW, Garg J, et al. Rivaroxaban versus warfarin in nonvalvular atrial fibrillation. *New England Journal of Medicine* 2011; 365: 883–891.

Evidence for the non-inferiority of apixaban compared to warfarin and aspirin for stroke and systemic embolism prevention in patients with non-valvular atrial fibrillation comes from the ARISTOTLE and AVERROES trials, respectively. See: Granger CB, Alexander JH, McMurray JJ, et al. Apixaban versus warfarin in patients with atrial fibrillation. *New England Journal of Medicine* 2011; 365: 981–992; Connolly SJ, Eikelboom J, Joyner C, et al. Apixaban in patients with atrial fibrillation. *New England Journal of Medicine* 2011; 364: 806–817.

---

## MICRO-facts

NICE guidelines recommend the use of rivaroxaban or apixaban in patients where warfarin use is not recommended and patients have one of the following risk factors:

- Congestive heart failure
- Hypertension
- Age 75 years or above
- Diabetes mellitus
- Previous TIA or stroke

National Institute for Health and Care Excellence. Atrial fibrillation: the management of atrial fibrillation. NICE guidelines [CG180]. London: National Institute for Health and Care Excellence, 2014.

---

Thrombolytic agents

| Mode of action: | CVS therapeutic use: |
|---|---|
| <ul><li>Streptokinase forms a complex with plasminogen, converting it to plasmin.</li><li>Alteplase, reteplase and tenecteplase are recombinant tPAs converting plasminogen to plasmin.</li></ul> | <ul><li>STEMI</li><li>Stroke</li><li>Life-threatening PE</li></ul> |

*Streptokinase, alteplase, reteplase, tenecteplase (IV administration)*

Side effects:

■ • Nausea and vomiting
■ • Bleeding (injection site, stroke) → Excess anti-thrombotic effect

Streptokinase

■ • Hypotension
■ • Anaphylaxis on repeat → Derived from streptococci, after a
  administration     first dose of streptokinase antibodies
           may be produced

Beware:

• Before thrombolysis in acute STEMI and stroke, check the list of absolute
  and relative contraindications before use of thrombolytics (see Section 3.4).

---

## MICRO-facts

*Veins:* slow-flow systems result in fibrin-rich clots (use anti-coagulants)
*Arteries:* fast-flow systems result in platelet-rich clots (use anti-platelets)

---

# 17.5 ANTI-PLATELET AGENTS

## PHYSIOLOGICAL BACKGROUND

Platelets are essential in ensuring haemostasis through a three-step process
(see Figure 17.6):

• *Platelet adhesion:* platelets adhere to the collagen in the subendothelium
  directly through glycoprotein GP Ia/IIb or through von Willebrand's factor
  (vWF) and glycoprotein Ib/IX/V.
• *Platelet activation:* platelets release dense and $\alpha$ granules containing various
  chemicals through exocytosis, including ADP, thromboxane ($TXA_2$) and vWF.
• *Platelet aggregation:* is achieved through the activation of glycoprotein
  IIb/IIIa that results in cross-links between platelets mediated by fibrinogen.

  • GP IIb/IIIa                    Inhibited by mono-
                       clonal antibodies

  The activation of GP IIb/IIIa results from a rise in intracellular calcium
  caused by:

  • ADP interaction with $P2Y_{12}$            Inhibited by clopidogrel
  • $TXA_2$ interaction with its receptor      Inhibited by aspirin
  • Thrombin (IIa) interaction with its receptor   Inhibited by some
                       anti-coagulants
  • Phosphodiesterase enzyme's action on cAMP   Inhibited by
                       dipyridamole

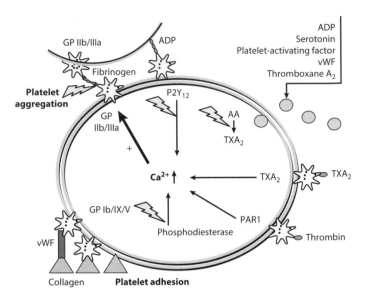

**Figure 17.6** Platelet clotting.

## Aspirin (acetylsalicylic acid)

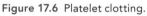

| Mode of action: | CVS therapeutic use: |
|---|---|
| • Inhibition of cyclooxygenase (COX) enzyme, reduces thromboxane ($TXA_2$) production from arachidonic acid (AA) in platelets. Reduced exocytosis and receptor stimulation increases cAMP and results in a fall in intracellular $Ca^{2+}$, not activating GP IIb/IIIa.<br>• Inhibition of cyclooxygenase in endothelial cells reduces prostacyclin production, reducing platelet aggregation, but the effect is very transient. | • ACS<br>• Primary and secondary prevention of ACS and TIA<br>• Analgesia<br>• Aneurysm prophylaxis in Kawasaki's disease |

Side effects:

■ • Gastrointestinal bleeding   →   Inhibition of COX-1 in the stomach decreases protective prostaglandin production that maintains the mucus layer

■ • Bronchospasm   →   Likely mediated from COX-1 inhibition leading to an increase in leukotriene levels

■ • Skin reaction   →   Hypersensitivity reaction

Cardiology and the cardiovascular system

Beware:
- Avoid in peptic ulcer disease, bleeding disorders, breast-feeding and hypersensitivity.
- Avoid in children below 16 years of age: Reye's syndrome (encephalopathy and liver disease).
- Irreversible inhibition of cyclooxygenase II means the effect of aspirin lasts for the duration of a platelet's life, 5–9 days.

## Thienopyridine
*Clopidogrel, prasugrel*

| Mode of action: | CVS therapeutic use: |
|---|---|
| • Irreversibly binds to P2Y$_{12}$ receptor, preventing ADP attachment. This inhibits the rise in intracellular Ca$^{2+}$ and subsequent GP IIb/IIIa activation. | • STEMI and NSTEMI<br>• Secondary prevention in STEMI and NSTEMI |

Side effects:
- Gastrointestinal bleeding    → Inhibition of platelet aggregation
- Abdominal pain/diarrhoea
- Nausea and vomiting

Beware:
- Avoid in active bleeding and breast-feeding.
- May lead very rarely to severe neutropenia and thrombocytopenic purpura (TTP).

## Ticagrelor

| Mode of action: | CVS therapeutic use: |
|---|---|
| • Similar to thienopyridines<br>• **Reversibly** blocks P2Y$_{12}$ receptors, preventing ADP attachment | • ACS<br>• Secondary prevention in ST segment elevation myocardial infarction (STEMI) and non-ST segment elevation myocardial infarction (NSTEMI) |

Side effects:

- ■ • Dyspnoea       →    Mechanism unknown – not caused by bronchospasm or reduced LV function
- ■ • Epistaxis and bruising
- ■ • Gastrointestinal haemorrhage
- • Intracranial haemorrhage
- • Dyspepsia, nausea, haematemesis

Beware:
- Avoid in active bleeding, previous intracranial haemorrhage and moderate-to-severe hepatic impairment.
- Avoid concurrent treatment with a strong CYP3A4 inhibitor (e.g. ketoconazole, clarithromycin) due to increased bleeding risk.

## Dipyridamole

| Mode of action: | CVS therapeutic use: |
|---|---|
| • Inhibits enzyme phosphodiesterase that is involved in cAMP hydrolysis. The rise in cAMP decreases $Ca^{2+}$, reducing activation of GP IIb/IIIa. | • Prosthetic heart valve<br>• Secondary prevention of transient ischaemic attack (TIA) and stroke |

Side effects:

- ■ • Gastrointestinal bleeding    →   Inhibition of platelet aggregation
- ■ • Headache, dizziness, hypotension, tachycardia, flushing    →   Effect of vasodilatation
- ■ • Diarrhoea

Beware:
- Avoid in active bleeding and breast-feeding.
- Avoid in unstable angina, aortic stenosis and hypertrophic cardiomyopathy because vasodilatory effects may aggravate the condition.
- May exacerbate migraines and myasthenia gravis.

## Glycoprotein IIb/IIIa inhibitors

*Abciximab (monoclonal antibody), eptifibatide, tirofiban*

| Mode of action: | CVS therapeutic use: |
|---|---|
| • Inhibit the GP IIb/IIIa, stopping cross-links forming between platelets and aggregation | • Prevention of ischaemia pre-percutaneous coronary angioplasty |

Side effects:

■ • Bleeding                         → Inhibition of platelet aggregation
■ • Nausea and vomiting
■ • Hypotension, bradycardia
■ • Thrombocytopenia

Beware:

- Avoid in active bleeding, recent intracranial trauma/major surgery/stroke, bleeding disorders.
- Avoid in breast-feeding.

---

**MICRO-case**

A 45-year-old man with new onset of atrial fibrillation was treated by electrical cardioversion and sinus rhythm was restored. After reviewing his history, comorbidities and his QT interval on ECG, the cardiologists recommended commencing amiodarone therapy. The patient underwent a baseline chest radiograph, U&E, thyroid and liver function tests. He was counselled on the risks of pulmonary fibrosis and ophthalmological complications and advised to look out for dyspnoea and blurred vision. The GP would subsequently monitor therapy by checking 6-monthly thyroid, liver and kidney function tests.

**Points to consider:**

- Counselling is essential prior to starting amiodarone due to the wide range of serious side effects it can cause such as pulmonary fibrosis.
- Patients need to be aware of the symptoms that might suggest thyroid disorder or pulmonary fibrosis.
- Patient should be warned about effects such as skin discoloration, which can be avoided with the use of sun screen.

Cardiology and the cardiovascular system

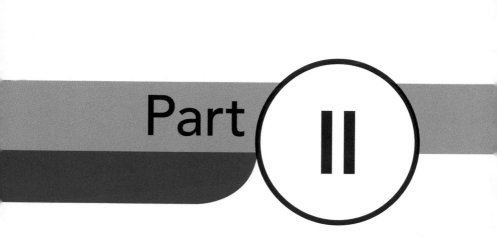

# Part II

# Questions and answers

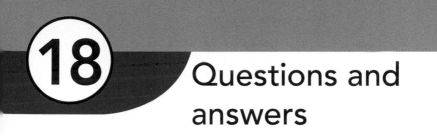

# Questions and answers

# Questions

## EMQs

For each of the following questions, please choose the single most likely drug responsible for the side effect. Each option may be used once, more than once or not at all.

## Pharmacology

- Amiodarone
- Bendroflumethiazide
- Clopidogrel
- Dipyridamole
- Flecainide
- Furosemide
- GTN spray
- Metoprolol
- Ramipril
- Simvastatin

### Question 1

A 45-year-old patient has attended the GP surgery complaining of a dry, irritating cough. His past medical history shows dyslipidaemia and recently diagnosed hypertension.

### Question 2

A 60-year-old active patient complains of recent-onset dry cough. In secondary care, pulmonary function tests reveal decreased carbon monoxide diffusion capacity. He has a past medical history of stable angina, hypertension, hypercholesterolaemia and atrial fibrillation.

## Question 3

A 62-year-old man attends the ED complaining of a swollen, red and painful big toe that appeared suddenly the night before. He had a previous episode many years ago. He tells you he has stable angina and high blood pressure.

**For each of the following questions, please choose the single most likely side effect of the drug mentioned. Each option may be used once, more than once or not at all.**

## Pharmacology

- Drug-induced lupus erythematosus
- Dry cough
- Dry mouth, urinary retention, raised intraocular pressure, constipation
- First-dose hypotension
- Gastrointestinal bleeding
- Nausea and vomiting, diarrhoea, yellow vision
- Optic neuritis
- Peripheral neuropathy
- Shortened PR interval
- Temporary flushing, sweating and dyspnoea

## Question 4

Hydralazine

## Question 5

Digoxin

## Question 6

Adenosine

**The following patients all present with acute heart failure. For each of the following questions, match the scenario to the likely aetiology.**

## Acute heart failure

- Aortic regurgitation
- Cardiac tamponade
- Constrictive pericarditis
- Ischaemic cardiomyopathy
- Mitral stenosis
- Myocarditis
- Papillary muscle rupture
- Pneumonia
- Pulmonary embolism
- Pulmonary fibrosis

## Question 7

A 60-year-old diabetic man is brought in by ambulance with new-onset severe shortness of breath. On examination, he is hypotensive and has a raised JVP. Auscultation reveals bilateral inspiratory crepitations and a harsh pansystolic murmur. The ECG in the ED shows ST segment elevation in leads II, III and aVF.

## Question 8

A 67-year-old hypertensive woman presents with sudden-onset stabbing anterior chest pain worst on inspiration. Her observations show tachycardia and hypotension and on examination she has a raised JVP, pulsus paradoxus and muffled heart sounds. Her ECG shows low-voltage complexes.

## Question 9

A 78-year-old breathless man is brought in by ambulance. His daughter has brought his medications, including a GTN spray, furosemide, ramipril and simvastatin. On examination, you find ankle oedema, raised JVP and bibasal inspiratory crepitations with coarse crepitations on the right side.

**For each of the following defects select the most likely underlying aetiology. Each option may be used once, more than once or not at all.**

## Congenital heart disease

- Congenital rubella infection
- DiGeorge syndrome
- Marfan's syndrome
- Maternal lithium use
- Maternal SLE
- Noonan's syndrome
- Prematurity
- Trisomy 21
- Turner's syndrome
- William's syndrome

## Question 10

A 6-month-old infant, with three previous admissions for chest infections, is under investigation for breathlessness, particularly when she eats. On examination, she is hypotonic, has wide epicanthic folds and a single palmar crease on each hand. She has an ejection systolic murmur heard at the upper left sternal edge and an apical pan-diastolic murmur. CXR shows increased pulmonary vascular markings and her ECG demonstrates a left axis deviation.

## Question 11

A neonate presents shortly after birth with signs of circulatory collapse. On a nitrogen washout test his oxygen saturations do not increase. The only pulse palpable is in the right arm. It is noticed that he also has a cleft palate and dysmorphic appearance.

## Question 12

A 6-year-old boy is complaining of chest pains when he runs. He is being seen for developmental delay and he appears to have unusual 'elfin' features. He is two standard deviations below the appropriate centile (on an age appropriate growth chart). On examination, he has an ejection systolic murmur heard at the upper right sternal edge.

**For each of the following presenting complaints, please choose the single most likely underlying congenital heart defect. Each option may be used once, more than once or not at all.**

## Congenital heart disease

- Aortic stenosis
- Coarctation of the aorta
- Hypoplastic left heart syndrome
- Persistent ductus arteriosus
- Pulmonary stenosis
- Tetralogy of Fallot
- Total anomalous drainage
- Tricuspid atresia
- Truncus arteriosus
- Ventricular septal defect

## Question 13

A patient presents at 5 months of age with worsening cyanosis. The parents report that this was not present at birth but developed in the last month. It is more pronounced at times, particularly when the child has been crying and at these times the infant appears to be in pain. There is a harsh ejection systolic murmur heard at the upper left sternal edge and a single second heart sound. On CXR, the heart appears to be 'boot shaped' and there are decreased pulmonary vascular markings.

## Question 14

A routine examination of a 5-month-old male infant reveals a continuous machinery murmur at the upper left sternal edge that radiates to the back. The infant is otherwise fit and well but required admission for a bronchiolitis infection previously.

## Question 15

A 15-year-old girl presents to her GP with short stature and delayed puberty. She is also found to have a harsh ejection systolic murmur that radiates through to her back. She has radio-radial and radio-femoral delay. Blood pressure is 170/98 mmHg in the right arm and 125/75 mmHg in the left arm.

**For each of the following questions, please choose the single most likely murmur. Each option may be used once, more than once or not at all.**

## Valvular heart disease

- Aortic regurgitation
- Aortic stenosis
- Flow murmur
- Mitral regurgitation
- Mitral stenosis
- Mitral valve prolapse
- Pulmonary regurgitation
- Pulmonary stenosis
- Tricuspid regurgitation
- Tricuspid stenosis

## Question 16

A 70-year-old woman presents with syncope on exertion and angina. On examination, she has a low volume pulse and an ejection systolic murmur heard over the right sternal edge that radiates to the carotids. Otherwise examination is normal. She had an MI 3 years previously.

## Question 17

A 40-year-old woman, who lived in Somalia until she was 25, presents with recurrent chest infections and haemoptysis. On examination, she has a pan-diastolic murmur heard at the apex, and left parasternal heave, a raised JVP and a tapping apex beat.

## Question 18

A 65-year-old man who was diagnosed with heart failure (secondary to ischaemic heart disease) 2 years previously has developed a new mid-systolic murmur on routine check-up. He has symptoms of breathlessness on exertion and orthopnoea. On examination, he also has a raised JVP and hepatomegaly.

For each of these cases select the most likely pathology. Each option may be used once, more than once or not at all.

## Valvular heart disease

- Amyloidosis
- Aortitis
- Calcific aortic stenosis
- Functional
- Infective endocarditis
- Ischaemia
- Mitral annulus calcification
- Rheumatic heart disease
- Rheumatoid arthritis
- Systemic lupus erythematosus

### Question 19

A 62-year-old man suddenly becomes breathless 24 hours after an MI. He had no prior history of cardiac disease. Echocardiography reveals regurgitation of the mitral valve.

### Question 20

A 54-year-old man begins to develop syncope and angina on exertion. Echocardiography reveals a bicuspid aortic valve.

### Question 21

A 42-year-old woman who had undergone a percutaneous mitral commissurotomy for rheumatic heart disease 3 weeks previously presents to her GP with malaise and a fever.

For each of the following cases select the most likely pathology. Each option may be used once, more than once or not at all.

## ECG and arrhythmias

- Anterior myocardial infarction
- Asystole
- Atrial fibrillation
- Atrial flutter
- Pericarditis
- Pulseless electrical activity
- SVT with bundle branch block
- SVT with normal conduction
- Torsades de pointes
- Ventricular fibrillation

- Ventricular tachycardia
- Wolff–Parkinson–White syndrome

## Question 22

An elderly patient presents with dyspnoea and palpitations. The ECG reveals regular broad complexes at a rate of 160 bpm. A review of his notes reveals previous ECGs with a similar QRS morphology (when he was in sinus rhythm and not tachycardic).

## Question 23

A patient is brought to the ED resuscitation area after a collapse. He has no pulse and demonstrates no respiratory effort. The ECG shows no evidence of identifiable atrial or ventricular activity.

## Question 24

You are called to an arrest on the orthopaedic ward. An elderly patient is found pulseless and with no respiratory effort but the ECG shows a heart rate of 40. She has recently undergone a total hip replacement.

**For each of the following cases select the most helpful investigation. Each option may be used once, more than once or not at all.**

## Investigation of chest pain

- Chest X-ray
- Coronary angiography
- CT chest
- CTPA
- ECG
- Endoscopy
- Exercise test
- Radionuclide bone scan
- Trans-oesophageal echocardiogram
- Transthoracic echocardiogram
- Troponin
- Ultrasound of the abdomen

## Question 25

A woman in her 50s is admitted with a 6-hour history of chest pain. She is also clammy and feels sick. Her past medical history includes diabetes and hypertension.

## Question 26

A 65-year-old man attends the ED with severe chest pain. The pain is noted to radiate between his shoulder blades. He has an early diastolic murmur and low blood pressure.

## Question 27

An elderly woman is readmitted with chest pain after a recent myocardial infarction (3 weeks previously) that was treated conservatively by optimizing drug treatment and no risk stratifying tests were done. Her ECG shows no acute changes and examination is unremarkable.

**For each of the following questions, please choose the single most likely diagnosis. Each option may be used once, more than once or not at all.**

## Examination of the JVP

- Acute ST elevation myocardial infarction
- Cardiac tamponade
- Complete heart block
- Congestive heart failure
- Constrictive pericarditis
- First-degree heart block
- Mitral regurgitation
- Superior vena cava obstruction
- Tricuspid regurgitation
- Tricuspid stenosis

## Question 28

A 65-year-old woman presents with a year long history of increasing pedal swelling and reduced exercise tolerance. She denies chest pain and risk factors for ischaemic heart disease. Her past medical history includes osteoarthritis and breast cancer treated aggressively 15 years ago. Clinically, she has pitting oedema bilaterally to her knees, a clear chest and normal heart sounds. Her JVP is raised at 5 cm above the sternal angle and appears to rise with inspiration. Echocardiogram shows good left ventricular function.

## Question 29

A 70-year-old man with known ischaemic heart disease presents to the ED with severe chest pain that had started 20 minutes ago and was radiating to the jaw. Initial observations reveal tachypnoea, a heart rate of 35 beats per minute and hypotension. Clinically, heart sounds are normal and the chest is clear. The JVP is visible and appears to have a very prominent first 'a' wave.

## Question 30

A 50-year-old man presents with 6 weeks of periodic chills, weight loss and bilateral ankle swelling. His past medical history is unremarkable aside from a hospital admission 2 years ago due to opiate overdose. On examination, he is mildly pyrexic with finger clubbing, marked pedal oedema and a heart murmur. His JVP is elevated and the double waveform is visible. The 'v' wave is especially prominent.

**For each of the following questions, please choose the single most likely diagnosis for the chest pain scenarios. Each option may be used once, more than once or not at all.**

## Chest pain

- Acute pericarditis
- Aortic dissection
- Aortic stenosis
- Musculoskeletal pain
- Myocarditis
- Non-ST elevation myocardial infarction
- Oesophagitis
- Pneumothorax
- Stable angina
- Unstable angina

## Question 31

A tall 40-year-old man comes to the ED complaining of dizziness and sudden-onset severe central chest pain radiating to the back. He has no past medical history of note and has never experienced chest pain before. Clinically, his pulse if regular, he is tachycardic and hypotensive. He appears to have a high-arched palate, central trachea, normal heart sounds, symmetrical chest expansion and normal breath sounds.

## Question 32

A diabetic 67-year-old woman on the orthopaedic ward experiences sudden-onset central chest pain that has lasted for 30 minutes. She has been receiving appropriate regular low-molecular-weight heparin. Clinical examination is unremarkable apart from a regular tachycardia. The ECG shows T wave inversion in leads II and III. Serial troponin measurements show no significant increase and her D-dimer is unremarkable.

## Question 33

A 78-year-old woman who lives alone presents to her GP surgery complaining of nausea and central chest pain occurring at rest over the past 3 months. Her background is unremarkable apart from osteoporosis and an older brother who has previously undergone a CABG operation. Her drug history shows she has recently been started on bisphosphonate therapy. At rest, her 12-lead ECG is normal.

For each of the following questions, please choose the single best next management step for the following cases of chest pain. Each option may be used once, more than once or not at all.

## Treatment of chest pain

- Antibiotics
- Chest drain
- Corticosteroids
- Valve replacement
- GTN spray
- Simple analgesia
- Low-molecular-weight heparin
- NSAIDs with proton pump inhibitors
- Percutaneous coronary intervention
- Warfarin

## Question 34

A 48-year-old man presents with 4 months of dull central chest pain and dizziness experienced upon exertion and relieved within minutes by rest. This is on a background of more long-standing shortness of breath and the man confides that he sleeps on three pillows. He denies having ankle swelling or any past history of heart attacks, diabetes or high cholesterol. Upon further enquiry he reveals that in the past he experienced a childhood febrile illness with joint pain.

## Question 35

A 60-year-old woman presents to the ED with shortness of breath and severe chest pain that has lasted an hour and remains unrelieved by her GTN spray. Her ECG shows a sinus tachycardia and T wave inversion in leads V1, V2 and aVF. Her serial troponins fail to show a rise over time. Her drug history includes simvastatin, chlorthalidone and ramipril. Her past medical history comprises angina, hypertension, systemic lupus erythematosus and recurrent miscarriages.

## Question 36

A 49-year-old woman returns to clinic 2 months after a myocardial infarction that had been treated by primary PCI. She has been experiencing chest pain over the past week relieved by sitting forward but not by using her GTN spray. The chest pain is associated with shortness of breath and chills. Clinical examination is unremarkable but the ECG shows ST segment elevation.

For each of the following questions, please choose the single most likely examination finding. Each option may be used once, more than once or not at all.

## Examination of the pulse

- Bradycardia
- Collapsing pulse
- Irregularly irregular pulse
- Pulsus alternans
- Pulsus bisferiens
- Pulsus paradoxus
- Radio-femoral delay
- Regularly irregular pulse
- Slow-rising pulse

### Question 37

An elderly patient presents with breathlessness and chest pain. On examination, there is a third heart sound and the JVP is significantly elevated; bibasal crepitations are elicited on auscultation.

### Question 38

A retired engineer presents with chest pain and breathlessness on exertion. On auscultation of his precordium, he has a harsh ejection systolic murmur radiating to the carotids.

### Question 39

A 30-year-old female attends an outpatient appointment with weight loss, agitation and poor sleep for the last 3 months. On examination, she is thin, has fine tremor and proptosis of the eyes.

For each of the following questions, please choose the single most likely diagnosis for the syncope. Each option may be used once, more than once or not at all.

## Syncope

- Arrhythmogenic right ventricular cardiomyopathy
- Autonomic neuropathy
- Complete heart block
- Congenital long QT syndrome
- Hypertrophic cardiomyopathy
- Left atrial myxoma

- Mitral regurgitation
- Paroxysmal atrial fibrillation
- Pulmonary embolism
- Vasovagal syncope
- Ventricular tachycardia

## Question 40

A 77-year-old woman has triple vessel coronary artery disease with poor left ventricular function. She suffered from a STEMI that led to a full thickness infarct of the left ventricle. She is admitted after a blackout and reports episodes of rapid palpitations.

## Question 41

A middle-aged diabetic patient complains of syncope and excessive sweating. He is under the care of the foot clinic for a number of diabetic ulcers and tells you his diabetic control has been erratic.

## Question 42

A 45-year old man has felt unwell for 1 year. He has been seen by neurology for two episodes of arm weakness that resolved within 1 day. He attends cardiology after a syncopal episode while gardening. He is noted to have clubbing of his fingernails and a mid-diastolic murmur.

# SBAs

## Question 43

A 73-year-old man attends his GP after episodes of 'fainting'. His ECG (see Figure 18.1) is shown below. What is the diagnosis?
- Complete heart block
- First-degree heart block

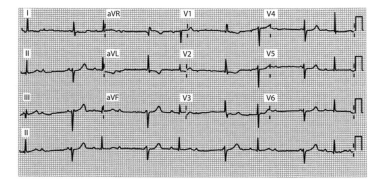

Figure 18.1 Question figure.

- Left bundle branch block
- Type 1 second-degree heart block (Wenckebach)
- Type 2 second-degree heart block

## Question 44

A 57-year-old male with dilated cardiomyopathy remains symptomatic in NYHA class II due to chronic heart failure. On examination, his pulse is 90 beats per minute and regular, BP is 140/90 mmHg and his heart sounds are normal. He is currently taking ramipril and furosemide. What is the next step in his medical management plan? Figure 18.2 shows his current ECG.

- Add amiodarone
- Add carvedilol
- Add digoxin
- Add spironolactone
- Increase furosemide dose

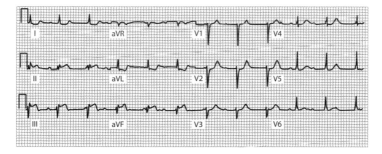

**Figure 18.2** Question figure.

## Question 45

You attend a crash call for an elderly patient on a medical ward. When you arrive nursing staff have started CPR and a monitor is attached. The rhythm is shown below in Figure 18.3.

What is the next step in the management of this patient?

- Defibrillation
- Further rounds of CPR
- IV adenosine

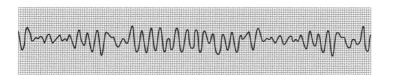

**Figure 18.3** Question figure.

- IV adrenaline
- IV amiodarone

## Question 46

An 80-year-old woman presents with severe chest pain radiating to the jaw. Her ECG in the ED is shown below. She is taken to the catheter laboratory for urgent PCI. Which region is affected by the infarct?

- Anterior
- Inferior
- Lateral wall
- Posterior
- Septum

## Question 47

A patient who was treated with primary PCI for a myocardial infarction 3 weeks ago re-attends with chest pain and shortness of breath. His chest radiograph shows bilateral pleural effusions. There is ST elevation on his ECG and a friction rub is heard. What has caused this?

- Acute myocardial infarction
- Dressler's syndrome
- Heart failure
- Occlusion of coronary stent
- Ruptured papillary muscle

## Question 48

This patient presents to his GP with palpitations that have occurred inter-mittently for a number of years. The ECG is shown below (see Figure 18.4). What is the diagnosis?

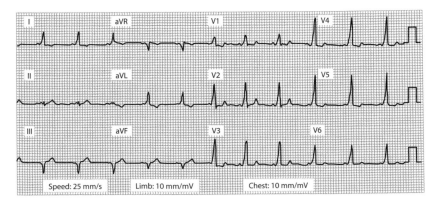

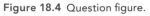

Figure 18.4 Question figure.

- Atrial fibrillation
- Atrial flutter
- AVNRT
- Ventricular ectopics
- Wolff–Parkinson–White syndrome

## Question 49

A 56-year-old male presents to the ED with palpitations. He has a history of IHD. His ECG is shown below (see Figure 18.5). What is the diagnosis?
- Atrial fibrillation
- Atrial flutter
- AVNRT
- Ventricular ectopics
- Wolff–Parkinson–White syndrome

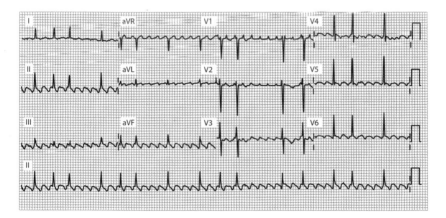

Figure 18.5 Question figure.

## Question 50

A young female patient presents to the ED with right-sided weakness and dysphasia that last 4 hours. She has just returned from a vacation in Australia. The CT head and ECG are normal, but the MRI head shows a small infarct. How should she be investigated further?
- Carotid dopplers
- Cerebral angiography
- Ultrasound scan of the carotid arteries
- Echocardiogram
- Coronary angiography

## Question 51

A neonate suddenly appears grey, with absent peripheral pulses 5 hours after birth. He is started on a prostaglandin infusion. Which of the following is mostly like to be a side effect of this?

- Apnoeas
- Hypoglycaemia
- Hypotonia
- Vomiting
- Worsening cyanosis

## Question 52

A 65-year-old man with a history of asthma and heart failure is admitted in new fast AF. He is given salbutamol to treat a wheezy chest and he is loaded with digoxin to slow his ventricular rate. His regular medications are continued. His bloods on day 2 show hypokalaemia. Which of his medications are likely to have caused this?

- Codeine phosphate
- Digoxin
- Ramipril
- Salbutamol
- Spironolactone

## Question 53

A 30-year-old male with hypertrophic cardiomyopathy presents in clinic with dizzy spells but has not had any syncopal episodes. Which of the following are indicators of increased risk of sudden cardiac death?

- A blood pressure drop during exercise
- Asymmetric septal hypertrophy with maximum wall thickness of 2 cm
- Left ventricular outflow tract gradient of 80 mmHg
- Systolic anterior movement of the mitral valve on echocardiography
- Worsening exertional angina

# Answers

## EMQs

### Pharmacology

### Answer 1

(**Ramipril**) Ramipril is an ACE inhibitor used frequently to control hypertension in patients under the age of 55 years (see Section 10.3 on hypertension). ACE is also the enzyme responsible for the degradation of bradykinins in the lung tissue, and accumulation of these with the use of ACE inhibitors leads to irritation and a dry cough. The cough may be irritating enough for patients to discontinue the medication, making it necessary to warn them of this side effect. For these patients, it is useful to consider an angiotenin II receptor blocker instead. Other common side effects of ACE inhibitors are dizziness and headache.

## Answer 2

(**Amiodarone**) Amiodarone is an anti-arrhythmic that can be used to maintain sinus rhythm in patients with atrial fibrillation episodes, especially in the presence of structural heart disease (see Section 14.1 on narrow complex tachycardia). Pulmonary fibrosis may occur in as many as 15% of patients on amiodarone, and results from the deposition of phospholipids within the alveolar macrophages and type 2 cells in the lung. The risk is higher for older patients on greater doses for a longer period of time. The CXR may demonstrate diffuse fibrosis, which may improve upon drug withdrawal.

## Answer 3

(**Bendroflumethiazide**) Bendroflumethiazide is a thiazide diuretic commonly used in essential hypertension as a first-line therapy (see Section 10.3 on hypertension). Thiazide diuretics can reduce uric acid excretion, precipitating acute gout in susceptible individuals. It may need to be withdrawn and replaced with another hypertensive. A calcium channel blocker, such as amlodipine, may be a solution and would also be useful for anginal symptoms. Other possible serum abnormalities with thiazide diuretics include hyponatraemia, hypokalaemia, hypercalcaemia and metabolic alkalosis.

## Pharmacology

## Answer 4

(**Drug-induced lupus erythematosus**) Hydralazine is an anti-hypertensive commonly used intravenously in pre-eclampsia and eclampsia of pregnancy. This agent is known to cause drug-induced lupus erythematosus if used long-term. This form of lupus erythematosus is caused by an autoimmune reaction precipitated by hydralazine and up to 5% of patients on long-term therapy may demonstrate this side effect. Other drugs known to cause lupus erythematosus include procainamide (class Ia anti-arrhythmic) and isoniazid (antibiotic). Other side effects of hydralazine include a tachycardia in response to systemic vasodilatation.

## Answer 5

(**Nausea and vomiting, diarrhoea, yellow vision**) Digoxin is an anti-arrhythmic drug used to control ventricular rate in sedentary patients with atrial fibrillation. Given its narrow therapeutic range, digoxin toxicity may be problematic.

Classic features include yellow and blurred vision, gastrointestinal disturbance and delirium. On the ECG, it is worth noting a prolonged PR interval and down-staging ST segment depression (reverse tick sign). Patients at risk include those on potassium-depleting diuretics because hypokalaemia potentiates digoxin effect. Overdose may be reversed using digoxin-specific antibody fragments.

## Answer 6

(**Temporary flushing, sweating and dyspnoea**) Adenosine is a drug given IV through a large-bore cannula to terminate paroxysmal supraventricular tachy-cardias. It also produces uncomfortable symptoms such as sweating, dyspnoea and flushing. Other side effects are lightheadedness and nausea and the patient may classically describe a 'feeling of impending doom'. These are secondary to the temporary asystole induced by adenosine before it is rapidly broken down in the circulation.

## Acute heart failure

### Answer 7

(**Papillary muscle rupture**) The man is likely to have had an inferior wall infarction leading to rupture of a portion of the posteromedial papillary muscle of the mitral valve. The result is hypotension and acute pulmonary oedema, with elevated atrial pressures and biventricular failure. Note the absence of pain, not uncommon in a diabetic patient.

### Answer 8

(**Cardiac tamponade**) The patient is likely to have developed a cardiac tam-ponade secondary to proximal aortic dissection. Hypertension is an important risk factor for this. Note that the anterior nature of the pain is plausible in light of ascending/aortic arch dissection.

### Answer 9

(**Pneumonia**) The most likely diagnosis is an acute pneumonia (as evidenced by the focal crepitations on auscultation). Infections commonly lead to decompensation in chronic heart failure. The list of medications suggests ischaemic heart disease as the aetiology of the chronic heart failure; however, this is not the cause of acute deterioration.

## Congenital heart disease

### Answer 10

(**Trisomy 21**) This patient has the symptoms and signs of a large primum ASD. She also has some of the features of Down's syndrome with which primum ASD (a type of AVSD) has an association.

## Answer 11

(**DiGeorge syndrome**) This patient has symptoms of either a coarctation of the aorta or complete interruption of the aorta. This is common in DiGeorge syndrome, which is also associated with a cleft palate, facial abnormalities, other heart defects (tetralogy of Fallot), thymic aplasia and hypocalcaemia.

## Answer 12

(**William's syndrome**) This patient has signs and symptoms suggestive of aortic stenosis. He also has signs of William's syndrome which is associated with supravalvular aortic stenosis.

## Congenital heart disease

## Answer 13

(**Tetralogy of Fallot**) This infant has a cyanotic heart defect; tetralogy of Fallot is the most common of the cyanotic heart defects. Depending on the severity it may not present at birth, as it may take time for a pressure gradient to develop and the pulmonary stenosis worsens with age. The periods of crying in which cyanosis worsens is a description of the 'hypercyanotic spells' characteristic of tetralogy of Fallot. The findings on examination and the investigations support this diagnosis.

## Answer 14

(**Persistent ductus arteriosus**) This patient has a murmur of a patent ductus arteriosus. As this is still present at 5 months, it is termed a persistent ductus arteriosus. These defects are often asymptomatic but a particularly severe respiratory infection may increase pulmonary blood flow.

## Answer 15

(**Coarctation of the aorta**) This patient has the signs and symptoms of a partial obstruction in the aorta. These defects can be asymptomatic but as she gets older she may develop hypertension, heart failure or arrhythmias. This patient also has delayed puberty and short stature, suggesting that she may need to be tested for Turner's syndrome, which is associated with coarctation of the aorta.

## Valvular heart disease

## Answer 16

(**Aortic stenosis**) This patient has the classic symptoms and murmur of aortic stenosis. She also has a history of coronary artery disease, which is frequently found concurrently with calcific aortic stenosis.

## Answer 17

(**Mitral stenosis**) This patient has a murmur suggestive of mitral stenosis and she has developed signs of pulmonary venous congestion and right ventricular failure. As she is young and has previously lived in a developing country as a child, rheumatic heart disease (which most commonly causes mitral stenosis) is the likely aetiology.

## Answer 18

(**Mitral regurgitation**) This patient has a murmur suggestive of mitral regurgitation. The mitral regurgitation may be a functional effect secondary to left ventricular dilatation.

## Valvular heart disease

## Answer 19

(**Ischaemia**) In this case, the cause of the acute valve dysfunction is likely to be papillary muscle rupture secondary to the MI.

## Answer 20

(**Calcific aortic stenosis**) This patient has the signs and symptoms of aortic stenosis. The most common cause of aortic stenosis is calcific degeneration, which occurs prematurely in bicuspid valves, as in this case.

## Answer 21

(**Infective endocarditis**) Heart valve surgery is a specific risk factor for infective endocarditis, so it should be considered in all patients presenting in this way. The history of fever and malaise suggests subacute bacterial endocarditis and is likely to be due to staphylococcal infection.

## ECG and arrhythmias

## Answer 22

(**SVT with bundle branch block**) This man is experiencing SVT with bundle branch block. His previous ECGs show he had a bundle branch block. The morphology of the QRS complex in V1 and V6 will help differentiate left bundle branch block from right bundle branch block. Remember that in the case of a left bundle branch block it is not possible to exclude an elevation or depression in the subsequent ST segment.

## Answer 23

(**Asystole**) This patient's ECG confirms that the patient is in asystole following their arrest. It is important to note that asystole and pulseless electrical activity (PEA) constitute non-shockable rhythms.

## Answer 24

**(Pulseless electrical activity)** The situation suggests pulseless electrical activity, also known as electromechanical dissociation. There is electrical activity but no blood is being pumped. The history suggests that this may be due to a pulmonary embolism.

## Investigation of chest pain

## Answer 25

**(ECG)** Given the presence of cardiovascular risk factors such as diabetes and hypertension, myocardial infarction should be the number one differential diagnosis. The ECG should be the first investigation in this woman as it may reveal ST segment deviation or T wave inversion as would fit a diagnosis of acute coronary syndrome. Blood tests for troponins may be necessary to confirm a diagnosis 6–12 hours after the onset of pain.

## Answer 26

**(CT chest)** The history suggests that this man may have an aortic dissection and his examination suggests possible secondary aortic regurgitation. He requires urgent imaging, of which a CT chest will usually be the most easily available and sufficiently sensitive. TOE and MRI may be the investigations of choice but are normally limited by their availability.

## Answer 27

**(Troponin)** This woman may now be suffering from angina after her recent infarction. However, it is important to exclude a further infarction by checking for a rise in troponin. As the previous infarction was more than 2 weeks before this event, troponin should have returned to baseline. She requires an angiogram to assess any coronary artery narrowing and to assess her suitability for intervention. In some individuals exercise testing, CT scans of the coronary arteries or perfusion scanning may also be an option depending on the predictive risk of having ischaemic heart disease (NICE guidelines).

## Examination of the JVP

## Answer 28

**(Constrictive pericarditis)** Raised JVP, pedal oedema and poor exercise tolerance in this patient suggest cardiac congestion. The lack of previous chest pain and risk factors for ischaemic heart disease makes ischaemia-induced heart failure less likely. A JVP that rises with inspiration is a positive Kussmaul's sign. Taken together with an insidious onset and possible chest exposure to radiotherapy for breast cancer treatment, this sign is suggestive of constrictive pericarditis. The differential diagnosis for a positive Kussmaul's sign includes cardiac tamponade and restrictive cardiomyopathy. The presence of normal heart sounds in this case makes cardiac tamponade less likely, although recurrence of malignant disease may present with pericardial effusions (uncommonly).

## Answer 29

**(Complete heart block)** The patient has risk factors for ischaemic heart disease and the acute episode sounds like a myocardial infarction. It is important to hone in on the profound bradycardia as it suggests the development of conduction system defects post-infarction. In this case, a heart rate of 45 beats per minute would fit with a ventricular rhythm. Prominent 'a' waves are suggestive of complete heart block, as they can be produced by atrial contraction against a closed tricuspid valve due to uncoupling of the cardiac cycle.

## Answer 30

**(Tricuspid regurgitation)** The key aspects to pick up in this presentation are the systemic symptoms and the signs that localize it to the cardiovascular system: cardiac murmur and pedal oedema. A prominent 'v' wave fits with a diagnosis of tricuspid incompetence leading to accentuation of the back-pressure effect of ventricular contraction on the JVP. This is likely secondary to valvular destruction. Given the time course of the illness, it is important to consider subacute bacterial endocarditis. A past history of opiate overdose suggests intravenous drug use, a risk factor for right-sided bacterial endocarditis. Subacute bacterial endocarditis is one of the few cardiovascular causes of finger clubbing, others being cyanotic congenital cardiac disease and atrial myxomas.

## Chest pain

## Answer 31

**(Aortic dissection)** This relatively young man appears to be haemodynamically compromised. With acute chest pain this may commonly be secondary to a pulmonary embolism, tension pneumothorax, arrhythmia, acute myocardial infarction or aortic dissection. The patient's age and appearance suggestive of Marfan's syndrome (tall with a high-arched palate) predisposes him to both a spontaneous pneumothorax and aortic dissection. The normal respiratory examination and severity of chest pain make the second option more likely.

## Answer 32

**(Unstable angina)** This chest pain history is very suggestive of an acute coronary syndrome. Increasing age and diabetes are important risk factors for ischaemic heart disease. The ECG shows evidence of ischaemia that may be localized to the inferior aspect of the myocardium. There is no evidence of ST segment elevation, and this may be either a NSTEMI or unstable angina.

The lack of a rise in troponin levels confirms this as unstable angina. Myocardial infarctions are commoner in the post-operative setting.

## Answer 33

(**Oesophagitis**) This chest pain history may sound like unstable angina at first and the lack of ECG abnormalities at rest would not preclude the diagnosis. However, the case highlights the importance of eliciting a drug history in patients with chest pain. Bisphosphonates should be taken with a large glass of water and the patient should be advised to sit upright for 30 minutes post-ingestion. Failure to follow the advice may result in severe oesophagitis.

## Treatment of chest pain

### Answer 34

(**Valve replacement**) This is a relatively young man without the usual risk factors for ischaemic heart disease. He presents with a classic triad of symptoms for aortic stenosis: angina-like chest pain, shortness of breath and dizziness. The lack of ankle swelling implies pulmonary congestion without congestive cardiac failure. It is important to note the childhood febrile illness with joint pain as it may have been an episode of rheumatic fever leading on to rheumatic heart disease, a major cause of aortic stenosis. Note that dizziness in aortic stenosis is a sinister sign with a large mortality rate in the absence of valve replacement.

### Answer 35

(**Low-molecular-weight heparin**) This woman has systemic lupus erythematosus and possibly antiphospholipid syndrome as suggested by the recurrent miscarriages. This predisposes the patient to venous thromboembolism events such as pulmonary emboli. For a patient with a high risk of pulmonary emboli, it is necessary to start low-molecular-weight heparins prior to ordering a CT pulmonary angiogram and starting warfarin therapy in confirmed cases. In high-risk patients, a D-dimer is not very useful as it is not diagnostic. The main differential diagnosis to consider is an acute coronary event in this patient as she has established ischaemic heart disease. Her ECG changes and troponin tests may be interpreted as either signs of RV strain consistent with a pulmonary embolus or unstable angina resulting in right-sided ischaemia.

### Answer 36

(**NSAIDs with proton-pump inhibitors**) This patient has Dressler's syndrome, an antibody-mediated condition that occurs 4–8 weeks after a myocardial infarction and results in pericarditis. Chest pain relieved by sitting forward is typical of pericarditis, which is also a differential diagnosis for ST segment elevation. Characteristically, the ST segment elevation is saddle-shaped. Treatment is supportive and relies predominantly on NSAIDs.

Questions and answers

## Examination of the pulse

### Answer 37

**(Pulsus alternans)** The patient is in acute heart failure and may have pulsus alternans. This is due to the failing heart giving alternating weak and strong beats, which lead to both large and small volume pulses in the cycle.

### Answer 38

**(Slow-rising pulse)** This man has features of aortic stenosis, which would give rise to a slow-rising pulse and narrow pulse pressure.

### Answer 39

**(Irregularly irregular pulse)** The patient has features of Graves' disease. Hyperthyroidism commonly causes atrial fibrillation that would give rise to an irregularly irregular pulse.

## Syncope

### Answer 40

**(Ventricular tachycardia)** This woman is at risk of ventricular tachyarrhythmias due to the damage to her heart and extensive scar tissue. The rapid palpitations may have been previous episodes of VT. She requires monitoring and ultimately may require an ICD.

### Answer 41

**(Autonomic neuropathy)** This man has autonomic features and his history of poorly controlled diabetes with diabetic neuropathy should lead to autonomic neuropathy as a diagnosis.

### Answer 42

**(Left atrial myxoma)** The patient has been experiencing transient ischaemic attacks on a background of illness. The ischaemia is the result of tumour embolisms entering the cerebral circulation. The examination findings are in keeping with this diagnosis as left atrial myxoma is one of the few cardiovascular causes of clubbing. Atrial myxomas may interfere with the movement of the mitral valve, leading to a diastolic murmur.

## SBAs

### Answer 43

**Type 2 second-degree heart block**
The ECG shows type 2 second-degree heart block. There are non-conducted P waves occurring without an alteration in the PR interval. Type 2 second-degree heart blocks may often occur with a set ratio of P waves to conducted

QRS complexes such as 2:1 or 3:1. This rhythm may progress to a complete heart block and the patient will require an implantable pacemaker. In this case, there is 2:1 block with junctional escape beats.

## Answer 44
**Add carvedilol**
Beta-blockers have been shown to improve mortality and quality of life in chronic heart failure. Most commonly used are bisoprolol and carvedilol. They should be avoided in the acute setting and started only once the patient's disease is stable. Spironolactone is indicated in NYHA class III and IV heart failure. Digoxin may be added once other medications have been trialled. The patient is not in acute heart failure (presenting with worsening fluid overload such as in acute pulmonary oedema) and is not on maximal medical therapy so increasing the furosemide dose would be of little benefit.

## Answer 45
**Defibrillation**
The patient is in VF. This is a shockable rhythm and according to RESUS Council guideline the treatment is defibrillation before continuing CPR. Adrenaline and amiodarone are indicated later in the algorithm. Adenosine is used in the management of bradyarrhythmias as it transiently slows down conduction at the AV node.

## Answer 46
**Inferior**
The woman is suffering from an inferior MI. A lateral MI would present with changes in leads I and V4–V6. Septal infarcts show changes mainly in leads V1 and V2. Posterior MIs are best seen with additional back leads but appear as ST depression in anterior leads with dominant R waves. Anterior MIs can present with changes across all the chest leads.

## Answer 47
**Dressler's syndrome**
The patient has Dressler's syndrome. This is a pericarditis occurring 3–6 weeks post-MI. It occurs due to an immunological response to heart muscle proteins following damage, and thus differs from post-MI pericarditis that is an inflammatory response to tissue damage in the days following infarct. Dressler's syndrome may also occur after cardiac surgery.

## Answer 48
**Wolff–Parkinson–White syndrome**
The ECG shows a slurred upstroke or 'delta' wave and a short PR interval. These occur due to rapid conduction through an additional conduction bundle. In this

case the bundle of Kent. The patient has Wolff–Parkinson–White syndrome and is at risk of supraventricular tachycardia and sudden cardiac death.

## Answer 49

### Atrial flutter

The ECG shows typical flutter waves. The man has atrial flutter most likely due to his previous IHD. He will require cardioversion back into a sinus rhythm. Often patients will progress and may eventually develop atrial fibrillation.

## Answer 50

### Echocardiogram

The history is suggestive of a deep vein thrombosis developing during a long-haul flight and passing from the venous circulation on the right side of the heart to the left side. The embolus will travel up the carotid circulation and result in a transient ischaemic attack. This is termed a paradoxical embolus and commonly occurs due to a patent foramen ovale. The investigation of choice is a transthoracic echocardiogram with bubble contrast (shaken saline used as a contrast). A trans-oesophageal echocardiogram may be an option if the transthoracic echocardiogram with bubble contrast is inconclusive.

## Answer 51

### Apnoeas

Apnoeas and bradycardia are side effects of a prostaglandin infusion. Other side effects such as jitteriness may be confused with hypoglycaemia. The prostaglandin infusion should improve any symptoms derived from the heart defect.

## Answer 52

### Salbutamol

Salbutamol is known to cause hypokalaemia as it shifts potassium intracellularly. For this reason, it is used in the management of hyperkalaemia. Spironolactone and ACE inhibitors commonly cause hyperkalaemia, whereas codeine phosphate does not cause electrolyte disturbance. Although digoxin does not affect potassium levels, low potassium levels make digoxin toxicity more likely and should be treated to prevent this.

## Answer 53

### A blood pressure drop during exercise

Hypertrophic cardiomyopathy leads to an increased risk of sudden cardiac death due to ventricular tachyarrhythmias. Five indicators of an increased risk of sudden cardiac death are:

- Syncope
- Family history of sudden cardiac death due to hypertrophic cardiomyopathy

- Ventricular wall thickness greater than 3 cm
- Blood pressure drop during peak exercise on stress testing
- Runs of non-sustained VT on 24-hour tape

Left ventricular outflow tract (LVOT) obstruction causes but does not predict sudden cardiac death. Systolic anterior movement of the mitral valve is often seen on echocardiogram and may contribute to the LVOT.

# Index